Easy Keto Cookbook 2021

A Tailor Made Ketogenic Diet Program
With The Best Recipes For Weight Loss,
Fight Diseases And Healthy Living

CONTENTS

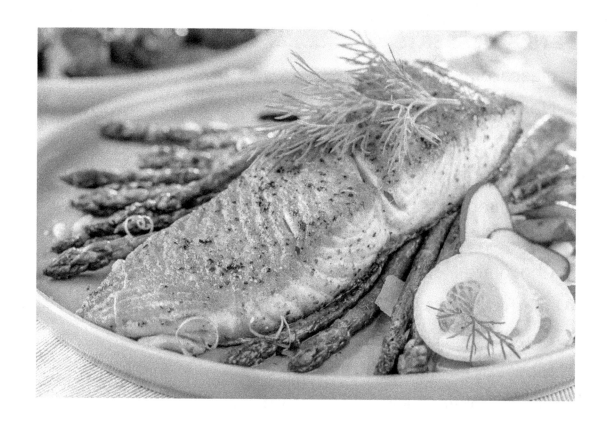

INTRODUCTION

It's widely-spread knowledge that our bodies are designed to run primarily on carbs. We use them to provide our bodies with the energy required to boost our state, exercise, or just normal body functioning. However, most people are clueless about the fact that carbs are not the only source of fuel our bodies can use. Just like they can run on carbs, our bodies can also use fat sources. When we ditch the carbs and focus on providing our bodies with more fat, we are embarking on the ketogenic train.

The ketogenic diet is not just another fad diet. It has been around since 1920 and has resulted in outstanding results and amazingly successful stories. If you are new to the keto world and have no idea what I am talking about, let me simplify this for you.

For you to truly understand what the keto diet is all about and why you should start it as soon as you can, let me first explain what happens to your body after consuming a carb-loaded meal.

Imagine you have just swallowed a giant bowl of spaghetti. Your tummy is full, your taste buds are satisfied, and your body is provided with more carbs than necessary. After consumption, your body immediately starts the process of digestion, during which your body will break down the consumed carbs into glucose, which is a source of energy your body depends on. So one might ask, "What is wrong with carbs?" For starters, there are some things: they raise the blood sugar, make your body work excessively to offset the effects of that sugar, and kindly storing it as another layer of fat, usually around the belly, but many times around the organs too. That's extremely dangerous. Sounds scary? I know.

By now, you've undoubtedly heard of the keto diet and the many people who have had success losing weight and keeping it off. But just what is a ketogenic diet, and how does it work to reach your weight loss goal.

The keto diet is a food plan that is high in fat and low in carbs. The human body uses carbohydrates as its primary fuel source; however, when fats replace carbs, the body enters a metabolic state known as "ketosis." During

ketosis, because of the lack of carbs, the body will burn stored fat as fuel, which can help you lose weight.

Not only can the keto diet promote weight loss, but it also comes with numerous health benefits:

- Management of diabetes
- Lower cholesterol
- Improved mental clarity
- Reduces the risk and symptoms of polycystic ovary syndrome (POS)
- Lower risk of some cancers
- Lower risk of cardiovascular disease

The keto diet requires a change in your wearing habits. It's easier to make these changes when you have your partner or other family members' active support. As a couple, you'll be able to encourage each other on those days that are more difficult than others for sticking to your food plan.

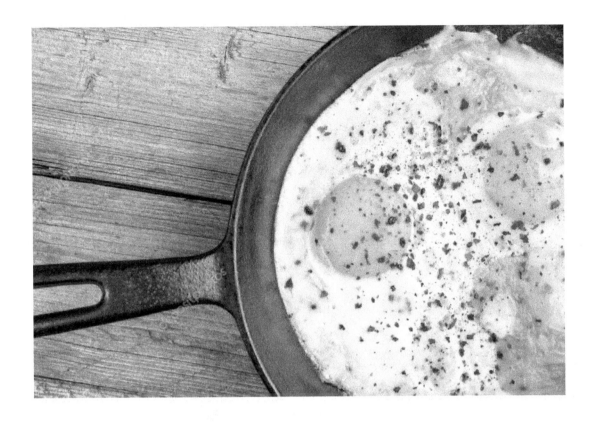

THE KETOSIS

Switching to high fat moderate protein cycle, your liver now has a new "fuel boss" - the fat. Once your liver begins preparing your body for the fuel change, the fat from the liver will start producing ketones – hence the name Ketogenic. What glucose is for the carbs, the ketones are for the fat, meaning they are the tiny molecules created once the fat is broken down to be used as energy. The switch from glucose to ketones is something that has pushed many people away from this diet. Some people consider this to be a dangerous process, but the truth is, your body will run just as efficiently on ketones as it does on glucose.

Once your body shifts to using ketones as fuel, you are in the state of ketosis. Ketosis is a metabolic process that may be interpreted as a little 'shock' to your body. However, this is far from dangerous. Every change in life requires adaptation, and so does this. This adaptation process is not set in stone, and every person goes through ketosis differently. However, for most people, it takes around 2 weeks to adapt to the new lifestyle fully.

Note! This is all biological and completely healthy. You have spent your whole life packing your body with glucose; naturally, you need time to adapt to the new dietary change.

Foods Allowed On the Keto Diet

Plan your meals and snacks around the following foods:

- Eggs
- Meats, including beef, pork, chicken, and veal
- Fish, including fish high in fat such as mackerel, trout, and salmon
- Cheeses
- Nuts and seeds, including nut and seed butter

10

- Cream and butter
- Avocadoes
- Healthy oils, such as olive, avocado, and coconut oils
- Low-carb vegetables, such as peppers, onions, tomatoes, and green vegetables
- Herbs and spices, including salt and pepper

To be sure you're getting enough of the right nutrients, eat a wide variety of meats, vegetables, seeds, and nuts on the allowed food list.

Foods Restricted On the Keto Diet

These are the foods that are restricted on a ketogenic food plan:

- Grains and starches, such as bread, pasta, cereal, and rice
- Carrots, potatoes, yams, sweet potatoes, and parsnips
- Beans and legumes, including chickpeas, lentils, and peas
- Fruit, except for small quantities of berries
- Sugar in any form, including foods that contain fructose
- Processed diet foods and Alcohol
- Condiments that contain sugar
- Unhealthy fats, such as processed vegetable oils and mayonnaise
- Alcohol

Getting Started with Your Keto Diet

Before starting the keto diet, take some time researching the foods on the allowed list and those restricted foods. Plan your meals ahead of time and shop accordingly, filling your kitchen with keto-friendly foods.

Healthy snacks

To make it easier to stick to the keto diet, it's important to have healthy snacks. If you're on the keto diet with your partner, have keto-approved snacks on hand that you both enjoy. Approved snacks include:

- Hard-boiled eggs, cheese, and olives
- A handful of nuts and seeds
- Celery and red pepper sticks with guacamole and salsa
- No-sugar plain yogurt mixed with berries

Intermittent Fasting and the Keto Diet

Intermittent fasting is all about restricting the number of calories you consume within a period so that you put your body into a "fasted" state. When this happens, the body's insulin levels will start to lower, which increases the fat burning process.

The Benefits of Intermittent Fasting Include:

- Weight loss
- Improved mental clarity
- Management and reducing the risk of type 2 diabetes
- Lower risk of cardiovascular disease
- Lower risk of some cancers

The most common fasting method is to fast each day for 14 to 16 hours, restricting the time you eat to a "window" of 8 to 10 hours. During the eating window, you should be eating at least 2 to 3 healthy keto meals. An excellent way to approach intermittent fasting is eating your last meal by 8 pm on any day and not eating your first meal until midnight the next day.

Another intermittent fasting method includes the 5:2 rule, where you only eat 500 to 600 calories per day on two days of the week, eating a healthy keto diet for the other five days. Another fasting method is the eat-stop-eat plan, where you fast for 24 hours twice a week.

Both intermittent fasting and the keto diet put the body into a ketosis state to use up stored fat for energy. When you combine intermittent fasting with the keto diet, you may be able to put your body into ketosis faster than dieting alone. This can lead to faster and more efficient weight loss.

What to Expect On the Keto Diet & Keto "Flu"

During the first few days of starting the Keto, you may experience an increase in hunger, lack of energy, and problems sleeping. Some people may also experience nausea and digestive issues.

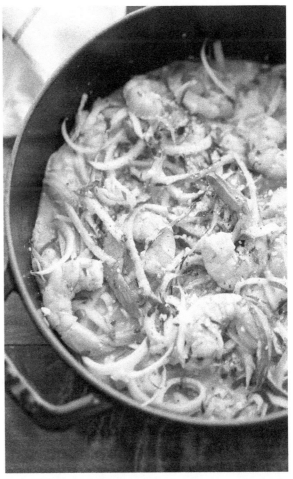

These flu-like symptoms are known as the "keto flu." To alleviate these symptoms, consider doing a low-carb diet for a week slowly transitioning into the full keto diet. During the first month, always eat until you feel full without focusing on restricting calories. Ease into the food plan, so you're less likely to stop eating a ketogenic diet.

The keto diet changes the mineral and water balance of your body. Make sure that you're drinking more water each day. As well, taking a mineral supplement and adding a bit of extra salt to your diet can keep help maintain a healthy balance of minerals and water, helping to relieve any of the flu-like symptoms. For a mineral supplement, take 300 mg of magnesium and 1,000 mg of potassium.

DIET – THE NEW LIFESTYLE

The Benefits of Keto Diet

Even though it is still considered 'controversial,' the keto diet is the best dietary choice one can make. From weight loss to longevity, here are the benefits that following a ketogenic diet can bring to your life:

Loss of Appetite

You can't tame your cravings? Don't worry. While on ketosis, you won't feel exhausted or with a rumbling gut. The keto diet will help you say no to that second piece of cake. Once you train your body to run on fat and not on carbs, you will experience a drop in appetite that will work magic for your figure.

Weight Loss

Since the body is forced to produce only a small amount of glucose, it will lower insulin production. When that happens, your kidneys will start getting rid of the extra sodium, which will lead to weight loss.

HDL Cholesterol Increase and Drop in Blood Pressure

While consuming a diet high in fat and staying clear of harmful glucose, your body will experience a rise in good HDL cholesterol levels, which will, in turn, reduce the risk for many cardiovascular problems. Cutting back on carbs will also drop your blood pressure. The drop in blood pressure can prevent many health problems such as strokes or heart diseases.

Lower Risk of Diabetes

Although this probably goes without saying, it is essential to mention this one. When you ditch the carbs, your body is forced to lower the glucose productivity significantly, which leads to a lower risk of diabetes, including a reverse in the condition if you already have it.

Improved Brain Function

Many studies have shown that replacing carbohydrates with fat as an energy source leads to mental clarity and improved brain function. This is yet another reason why you should go Keto.

Should You Try the Keto Diet?

The keto diet can help you lose weight and keep it off. When you're eating nutritiously, exercising, and following a ketogenic food plan, you'll be joining the many other people around the world who have successfully lost weight.

Whether you're starting the keto diet on your own or as a couple, begin with the keto food plan basics to become familiar with the foods you can and can't eat. As you start to lose weight and learn how to customize your meals, the keto diet plan will become a natural part of your lifestyle, allowing you to maintain your health and weight loss.

BASIC & SIMPLE RECIPES

1.AVOCADO BOATS WITH BACON & EGGS

Ingredients

For 4 servings

- 4 eggs

- 2 avocados, halved and pitted

- 2 bacon slices, chopped

- 2 tbsp chives, chopped

- 1 tsp smoked paprika

- Salt and black pepper to taste

Directions

Total Time: approx. 25 minutes

1. Preheat the oven to 360 F.

2. Scoop out some of the avocado flesh into a bowl.

3. Place the avocado halves in a greased baking dish and crack an egg into each half.

4. Season with paprika, salt, and black pepper and sprinkle with bacon.

5. Bake for 14-16 minutes or until set.

6. Top with fresh chives and serve.

Per serving:

- Cal 319

- Fat 28g

- Net Carbs 0.8g

- Protein 11 g

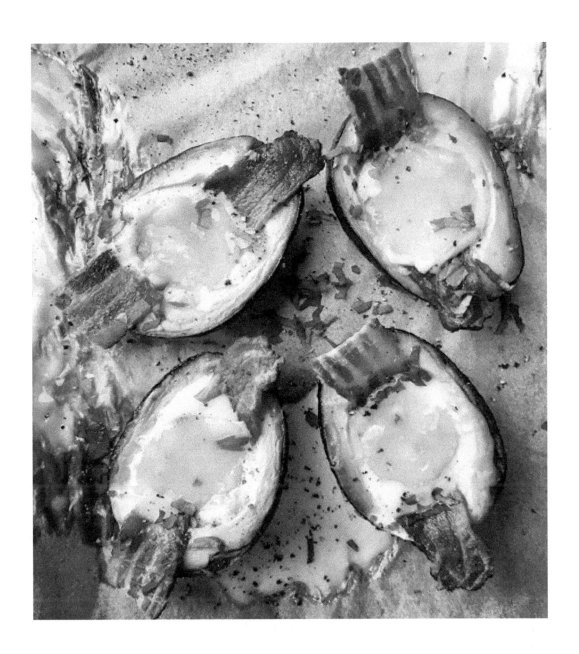

2.AVOCADO FRIES WITH CHIPOTLE MAYO SAUCE

Ingredients

For 4 servings

- 1 avocados, sliced
- 1 cup almond flour
- ¼ cup olive oil
- 1 tbsp lemon juice
- 2 large eggs, beaten
- 2 chipotle sauce
- ½ cup mayonnaise
- Salt and black pepper to taste

Directions

Total Time: approx. 20 minutes

1. Mix the almond flour with salt and black pepper.
2. Toss avocado slices in the eggs and then dredge in the flour mixture.
3. Heat olive oil in a deep pan and fry the avocado slices until golden brown, 2-3 minutes per side.
4. In a bowl, mix the mayonnaise, chipotle sauce, lemon juice, and salt.
5. Serve the fries with the sauce.

Per serving:

- Cal 633

- Net Carbs 2.7g
- Fat 58g
- Protein 11g

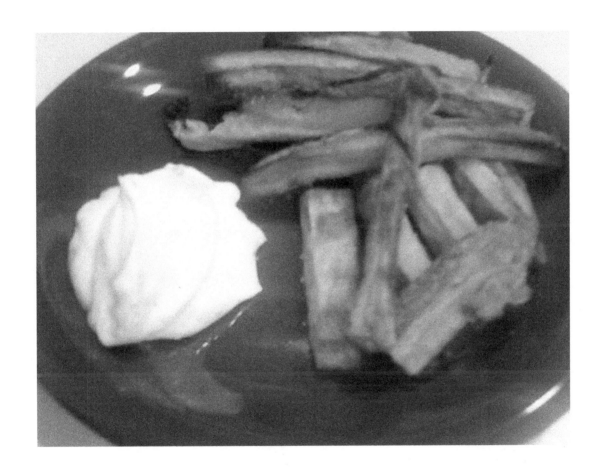

BREAKFAST
& EGGS

3. BELGIUM WAFFLES WITH CHEESE SPREAD

Ingredients

For 2 servings

- ½ cup cream cheese, softened
- 1 lemon, zested and juiced
- 2 tbsp liquid stevia
- 2 tbsp olive oil
- ½ cup almond milk
- 2 eggs
- ½ cup almond flour

Directions

Total Time: approx. 25 minutes

1. In a bowl, combine the cream cheese, lemon juice, lemon zest, and stevia.
2. In a separate bowl, whisk the olive oil, almond milk, and eggs.
3. Stir in almond flour and combine until no lumps exist.
4. Let the batter sit for 5 minutes to thicken.
5. Spritz a waffle iron with a cooking spray.
6. Ladle a ¼ cup of the batter into the waffle iron and cook for about 5 minutes.
7. Repeat with the remaining batter.
8. Slice the waffles into quarters; apply the lemon spread in between each of two waffles, snap, and serve.

Per serving:

- Cal 322
- Fat 26g
- Net Carbs 7.7g
- Protein 11g

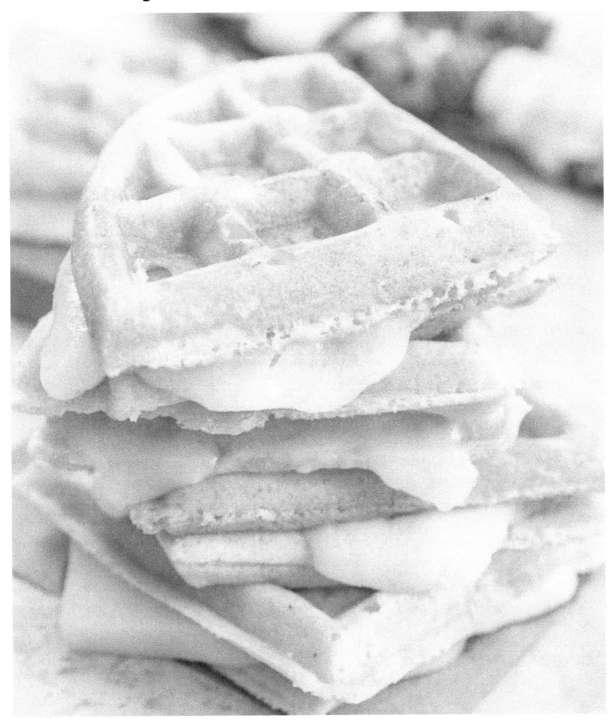

4. SPINACH & FETA CHEESE PANCAKES

Ingredients

For 2 servings

- ½ cup almond flour

- ½ tsp baking powder

- ½ cup feta cheese, crumbled

- ½ cup spinach, chopped

- 2 tbsp coconut milk

- 1 egg, beaten

Directions

Total Time: approx. 20 minutes

- In a medium bowl, put the egg, almond flour, baking powder, feta, coconut milk, and spinach and whisk to combine.

- Set a skillet over medium heat for a minute.

- Fetch a soup spoonful of the mixture and cook for 2 minutes.

- Flip the pancake and cook further for 1 minute.

- Remove onto a plate and repeat the cooking process until the batter is exhausted.

- Serve with your favorite topping.

Per serving:

- Cal 412

- Fat 32g

- Net Carbs 5.9g

- Protein 12g

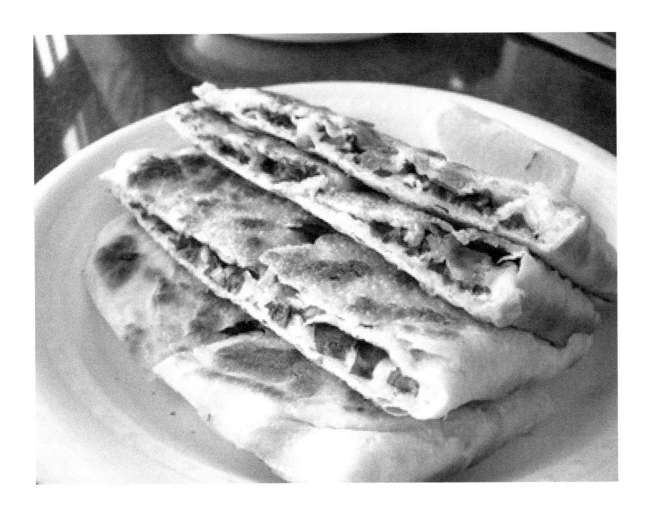

5. JALAPENO WAFFLES WITH BACON & AVOCADO

Ingredients

For 2 servings

- 1 tbsp butter, melted
- ¼ cup almond milk
- 2 tbsp almond flour
- Salt and black pepper to taste
- ½ tsp parsley, chopped
- ½ jalapeño pepper, minced
- 4 eggs
- ½ cup cheddar, crumbled
- 4 slices bacon, chopped
- 1 avocado, sliced

Directions

Total Time: approx. 20 minutes

1. In a skillet over medium heat, fry the bacon until crispy, about 5 minutes.
2. Remove to a plate.
3. In a bowl, combine the remaining ingredients, except for the avocado.
4. Preheat waffle iron and grease with cooking spray.
5. Pour in the batter and close the lid.

6. Cook for 5 minutes or until the desired consistency is reached.

7. Do the same with the rest of the batter.

8. Top with avocado and bacon.

Per serving:

- Cal 771
- Fat 67g
- Net Carbs 6.9g
- Protein 27g

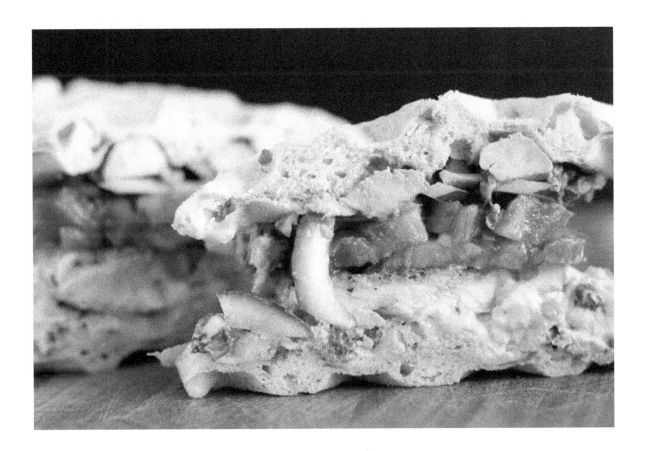

SALADS & SOUPS

6. SPINACH & BRUSSELS SPROUT SALAD

Ingredients

For 2 servings

- 1 lb Brussels sprouts, halved
- 2 tbsp olive oil
- Salt and black pepper to taste
- 1 tbsp balsamic vinegar
- 2 tbsp extra virgin olive oil
- 1 cup baby spinach
- 1 tbsp Dijon mustard
- ½ cup hazelnuts

Directions

Total Time: approx. 35 minutes

1. Preheat oven to 400 F.
2. Drizzle the Brussels sprouts with olive oil, sprinkle with salt and pepper, and spread on a baking sheet.
3. Bake until tender, 20 minutes, tossing often.
4. In a dry pan over medium heat, toast the hazelnuts for 2 minutes, cool, and then chop into small pieces.
5. Transfer the Brussels sprouts to a salad bowl and add the baby spinach.
6. Mix until well combined. In a small bowl, combine vinegar, mustard, and olive oil.
7. Drizzle the dressing over the salad and top with hazelnuts to serve.

Per serving:

- Cal 511
- Fat 43g
- Net Carbs 9.6g
- Protein 14g

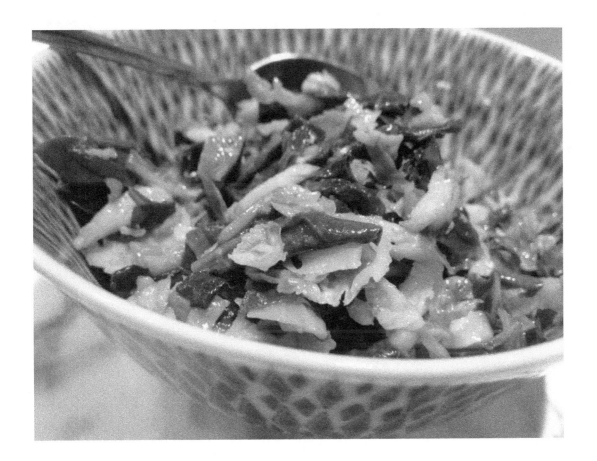

7. CHICKEN SALAD WITH PARMESAN

Ingredients

For 2 servings

- ½ lb chicken breasts, sliced
- ¼ cup lemon juice
- 2 garlic cloves, minced
- 2 tbsp olive oil
- 1 romaine lettuce, shredded
- 3 Parmesan crisps
- 2 tbsp Parmesan, grated

Dressing

- 2 tbsp extra virgin olive oil
- 1 tbsp lemon juice
- Salt and black pepper to taste

Directions

Total Time: approx. 30 min + chilling time

1. In a Ziploc bag, put the chicken, lemon juice, oil, and garlic.
2. Seal the bag, shake to combine, and refrigerate for 1 hour.
3. Preheat the grill to medium heat and grill the chicken for about 2-3 minutes per side.
4. Combine the dressing ingredients in a small bowl and mix well.
5. On a serving platter, arrange the lettuce and Parmesan crisps.

6. Scatter the dressing over and toss to coat.

7. Top with the chicken and Parmesan cheese to serve.

Per serving:

- Cal 529
- Fat 36g
- Net Carbs 4.3g
- Protein 34g

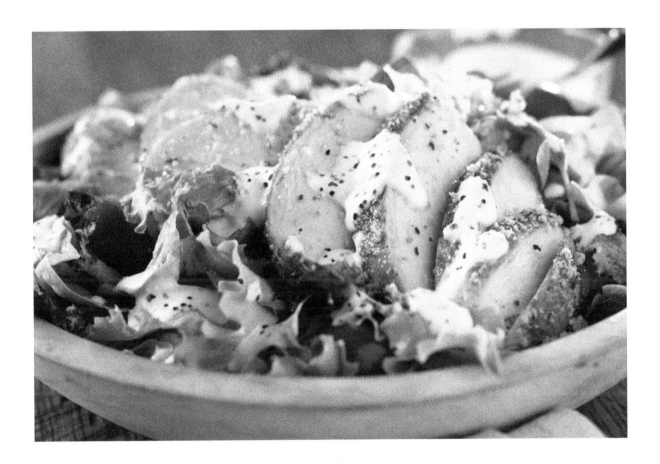

8. SMOKED MACKEREL LETTUCE CUPS

Ingredients

For 2 servings

- ½ head Iceberg lettuce, firm leaves removed for cups
- 4 oz smoked mackerel, flaked
- Salt and black pepper to taste
- 2 eggs
- 1 tomato, seeded, chopped
- 2 tbsp mayonnaise
- ¼ red onion, sliced
- 1 tsp lemon juice
- 1 tbsp chives, chopped

Directions

Total Time: approx. 20 minutes

1. Boil the eggs in a small pot with salted water for 10 minutes.
2. Then, run the eggs in cold water, peel, and chop into small pieces.
3. Transfer them to a salad bowl.
4. Add in the smoked mackerel, red onion, and tomato and mix evenly with a spoon.
5. Mix the mayonnaise, lemon juice, salt, and pepper in a small bowl and stir to combine. Lay two lettuce leaves each as cups and divide the salad mixture between them.
6. Sprinkle with chives and serve.

Per serving:

- Cal 314
- Fat 25g
- Net Carbs 3g
- Protein 16g

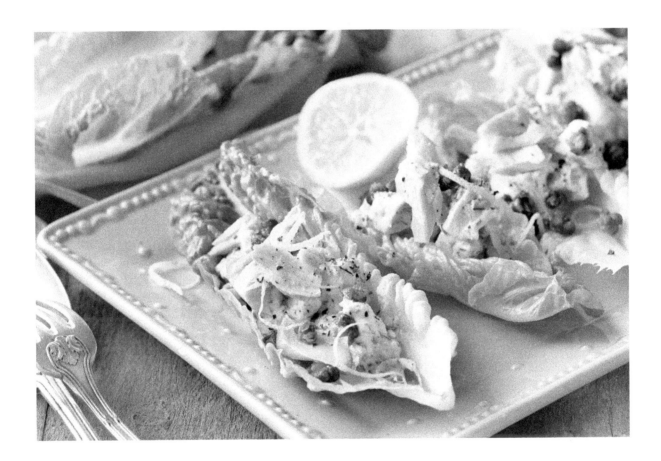

POULTRY

9. CHEESE & MAYO TOPPED CHICKEN BAKE

Ingredients

For 4 servings

- ½ cup Grana Padano cheese, grated
- 2 tbsp butter, melted
- 1 lb chicken breasts, halved
- Salt and black pepper, to taste
- ¼ cup green chilies, chopped
- 1 oz bacon, chopped
- 1 cup cottage cheese
- ½ cup mayonnaise
- 1 cup cheddar cheese, grated
- ¼ cup pork skins, crushed
- 2 tbsp basil, chopped

Directions

Total Time: approx. 55 minutes

- Preheat oven to 420 F.
- Coat the chicken with salt and black pepper and place in a greased baking dish.
- Pour in ½ cup of water and bake for 30 minutes.
- Cook the bacon in a pan over medium heat for 5 minutes until crispy.
- Remove to a bowl and let cool for few minutes.

- Stir in cottage cheese, ½ cup Grana Padano cheese, mayonnaise, chilies, and cheddar cheese.

- Spread the mixture over the chicken.

- Drizzle the melted butter over and sprinkle with the pork skins and remaining Grana Padano cheese.

- Bake in the oven for 5-10 minutes.

- Top with basil to serve.

Per serving:

- Cal 383

- Fat 21g

- Net Carbs 4.9g

- Protein 2g

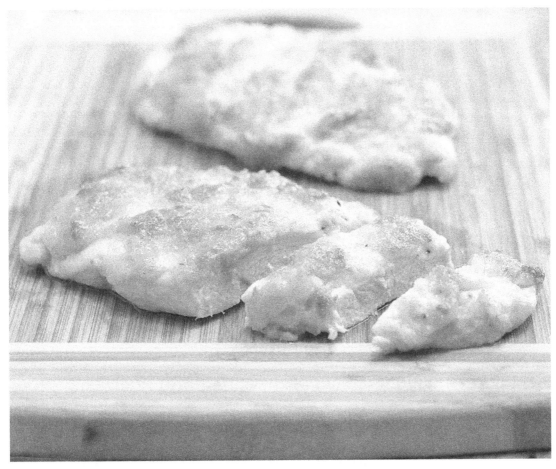

10. CHICKEN & SAUSAGE GUMBO

Ingredients

For 4 servings

- 1 sausage, sliced
- 2 chicken breasts, cubed
- 1 stick celery, chopped
- 1 bay leaf
- 1 bell pepper, chopped
- 1 onion, chopped
- 1 cup tomatoes, chopped
- 4 cups chicken broth
- 2 tbsp garlic powder
- 2 tbsp dry mustard
- 1 tbsp chili powder
- Salt and black pepper, to taste
- 1 tbsp cajun seasoning
- 2 tbsp olive oil
- 1 tbsp sage, chopped

Directions

- Total Time: approx. 40 minutes
- Heat olive oil in a saucepan over medium heat.
- Add the sausage and chicken and cook for 5 minutes.
- Add the remaining ingredients, except for the sage, and bring to a boil. Simmer for 25 minutes.

- Serve sprinkled with sage.

Per serving:

- Cal 433
- Fat 26g
- Net Carbs 8.7g
- Protein 36g

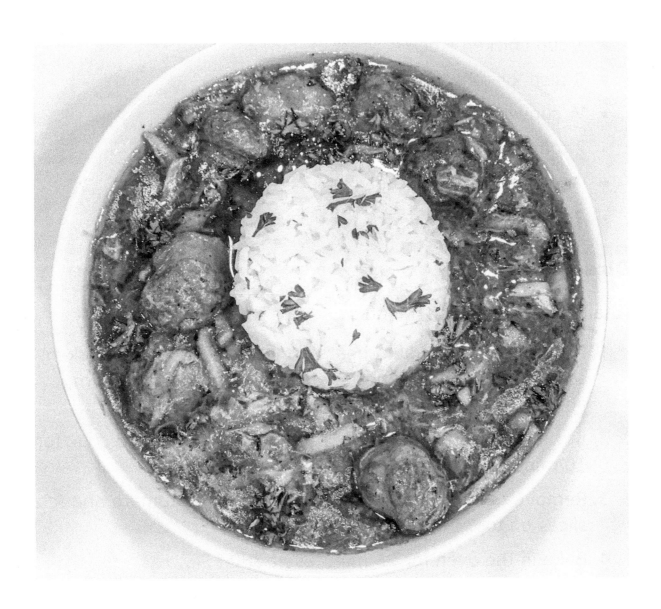

11. GREEK-STYLE BAKED CHICKEN

Ingredients

For 4 servings

- 1 tbsp olive oil
- 1 lb chicken breast halves
- 2 garlic cloves, minced
- Salt and black pepper, to taste
- 1 cup chicken stock
- 3 tbsp xylitol
- ½ cup white wine
- 2 tomatoes, sliced
- 4 oz feta cheese, sliced
- 2 tbsp dill, chopped

Directions

Total Time: approx. 40 minutes

1. Put a pan over medium heat and warm oil, add the chicken, season with black pepper and salt, and cook until brown, about 4-6 minutes.
2. Stir in the xylitol, garlic, stock, and white wine, and cook for 10 minutes.
3. Remove to a lined baking sheet and arrange tomato and feta slices on top.
4. Bake in the oven for 15 minutes at 380 F.
5. Sprinkle with chopped dill and serve.

Per serving:

- Cal 322
- Fat 15g
- Net Carbs 3.4g
- Protein 26g

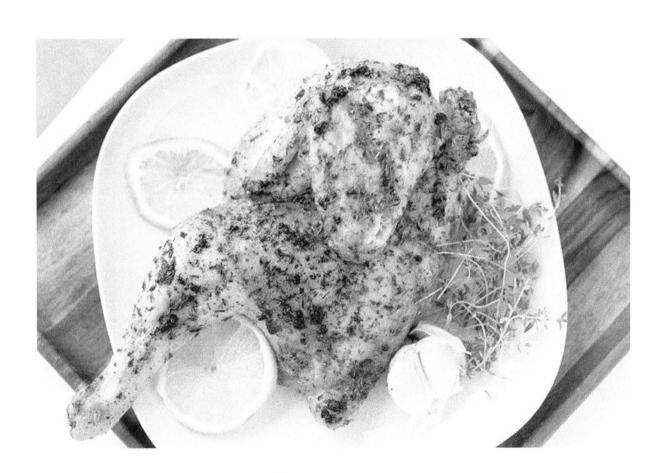

12. MEDITERRANEAN CHICKEN

Ingredients

For 4 servings

- 2 tbsp olive oil
- 1 onion, chopped
- 4 chicken breasts
- 4 garlic cloves, minced
- Salt and black pepper, to taste
- 10 Kalamata olives, chopped
- 1 tbsp capers
- 1 tbsp oregano
- ¼ cup white wine
- 1 cup tomatoes, chopped
- ½ tsp red chili flakes

Directions

Total Time: approx. 35 minutes

1. Brush the chicken with half of the olive oil and sprinkle with black pepper and salt.
2. Heat a pan over high heat and cook the chicken for 2 minutes, flip to the other side, and cook for 2 more minutes.
3. Transfer to a baking dish, add in the white wine and 2 tbsp of water.
4. Bake in the oven at 380 F for 1015 minutes.
5. Remove to a serving plate.

6. In the same pan, warm the remaining oil over medium heat.

7. Place in the onion, olives, capers, garlic, oregano, and chili flakes and cook for 1 minute.

8. Stir in the tomatoes, black pepper, and salt and cook for 2 minutes.

9. Sprinkle the sauce over the chicken breasts and serve.

Per serving:

- Cal 365
- Fat 22g
- Net Carbs 3.1g
- Protein 23g

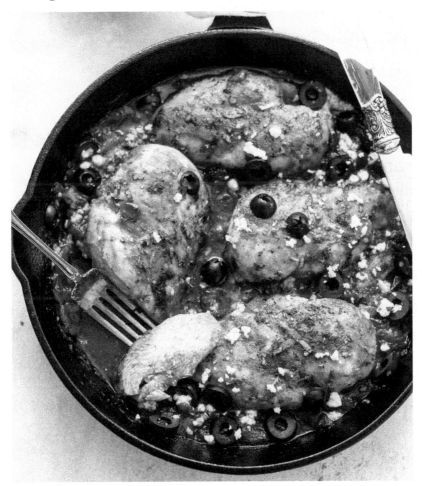

13. OVEN-BAKED SALAMI & CHEDDAR CHICKEN

Ingredients

For 4 servings

- 1 tbsp olive oil
- 1 ½ cups canned tomato sauce
- 1 lb chicken breasts, halved
- Salt and black pepper, to taste
- 1 tsp dried oregano
- 4 oz cheddar cheese, sliced
- 1 tsp garlic powder
- 2 oz salami, sliced

Directions

Total Time: approx. 40 minutes

1. Preheat oven to 380 F.
2. In a bowl, combine oregano, garlic, salt, and pepper.
3. Rub the chicken with the mixture.
4. Heat a pan with the olive oil over medium heat, add in the chicken and cook each side for 2 minutes.
5. Remove to a baking dish.
6. Top with the cheddar cheese, pour the tomato sauce over, and arrange the salami slices on top.
7. Bake for 30 minutes.
8. Serve warm and enjoy!

Per serving:

- Cal 417
- Fat 25g
- Net Carbs 5.2g
- Protein 29g

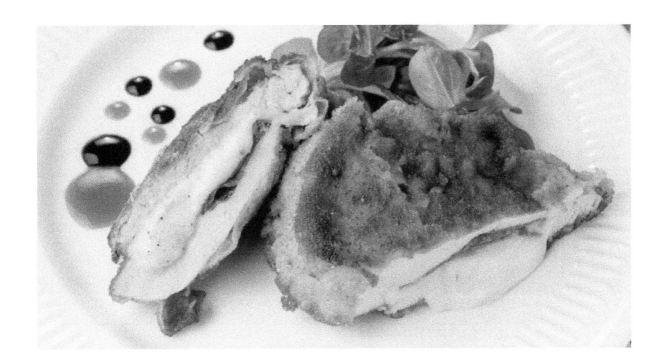

14. HAM & EMMENTAL BAKED CHICKEN

Ingredients

For 4 servings

- 1 lb chicken breasts, halved
- Salt and black pepper, to taste
- ¼ cup mayonnaise
- 1 tbsp Dijon mustard
- ¼ tsp xylitol
- ¼ cup pork rinds, crushed
- ¼ cup mozzarella, grated
- ¼ tsp garlic powder ¼ tsp onion powder
- Salt and black pepper
- 4 oz ham, sliced
- 2 oz Emmental cheese, sliced

Directions

Total Time: approx. 45 minutes

1. Preheat oven to 350 F.
2. Season the chicken with garlic and onion powders, salt and pepper.
3. In a bowl, mix mustard, mayonnaise, and xylitol.
4. Take about ¼ of this mixture and spread over the chicken.
5. Reserve the rest.
6. Spread half of the pork rinds and half of the mozzarella cheese on the bottom of a greased baking dish.
7. Place the chicken on top.
8. Sprinkle with the remaining mozzarella cheese and pork rinds.

9. Bake in the oven for about 25-30 minutes until the chicken is cooked completely.

10. Take out from the oven and top with Emmental cheese and ham.

11. Return to the oven and cook until golden brown.

12. Serve warm. Enjoy!

Per serving:

- Cal 443
- Fat 32g
- Net Carbs 5.1g
- Protein 31g

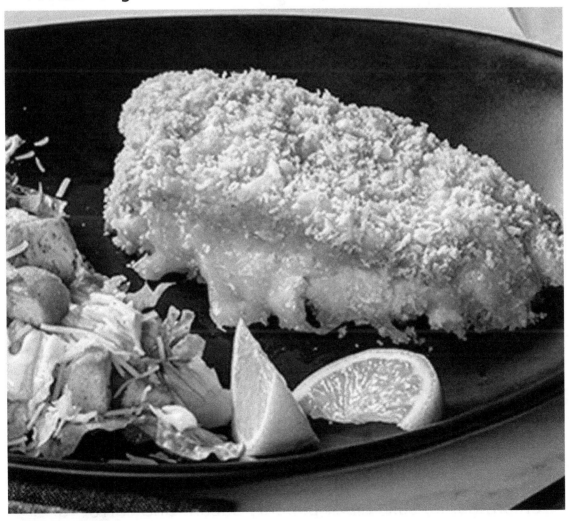

15. CHICKEN PIE WITH BACON

Ingredients

For 4 servings

- 3 tbsp butter
- 1 onion, chopped
- 4 oz bacon, sliced
- 1 carrot, chopped
- 3 garlic cloves, minced
- Salt and black pepper, to taste
- ¾ cup crème fraîche ½ cup chicken stock
- 1 lb chicken breasts, cubed
- 2 tbsp yellow mustard
- ¾ cup cheddar, shredded **Dough**
- 1 egg
- ¾ cup almond flour
- 3 tbsp cream cheese
- 1 ½ cups mozzarella, shredded
- 1 tsp onion powder
- Salt and black pepper, to taste

Directions

Total Time: approx. 50 minutes

1. Melt the butter in a pan over medium heat and sauté the onion, garlic, salt, black pepper, bacon, and carrot for 5 minutes.

52

2. Add in the chicken and cook for 3 minutes.

3. Stir in the crème fraîche, salt, mustard, black pepper, and stock and cook for 7 minutes.

4. Stir in the cheddar cheese.

5. For the dough, combine mozzarella and cream cheeses and heat in a microwave for 1 minute.

6. Stir in salt, almond flour, black pepper, onion powder, and egg.

7. Knead the dough well, split into pieces, and flatten into circles.

8. Set the mixture into ramekins, top with dough circles; cook in the oven at 370 F for 25 minutes.

Per serving:

- Cal 563
- Fat 44g
- Net Carbs 7.7g
- Protein 36g

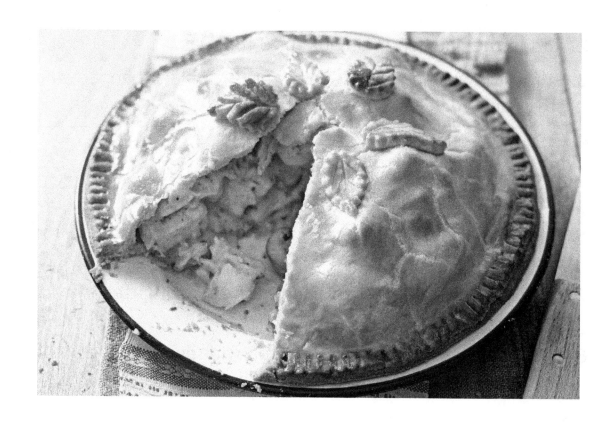

16. CAULIFLOWER & CHICKEN STIR-FRY

Ingredients

For 4 servings

- 1 large head cauliflower, cut into florets
- 2 chicken breasts, sliced
- 2 tbsp olive oil
- 1 red bell pepper, diced
- 1 yellow bell pepper, diced
- 3 tbsp chicken broth
- 2 tbsp chopped parsley

Directions

Total Time: approx. 25 minutes

1. Warm olive oil in a skillet and brown the chicken until brown on all sides, 8 minutes.
2. Transfer to a plate.
3. Pour bell peppers into the pan and sauté until softened, 5 minutes.
4. Add in cauliflower and broth and stir.
5. Cover the pan and cook for 5 minutes or until cauliflower is tender.
6. Mix in chicken and parsley.
7. Serve immediately.

Per serving:

- Cal 339

- Net Carbs 3.5g
- Fat 21g
- Protein 32g

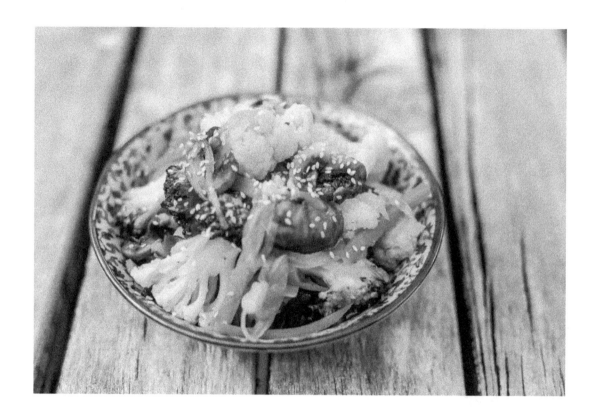

17. CREAMY MUSHROOM & WHITE WINE CHICKEN

Ingredients

For 4 servings

- 1 tbsp butter
- 1 tbsp olive oil
- 1 lb chicken breasts, cubed
- Salt and black pepper to taste
- 1 packet onion soup mix
- 2 cups chicken broth
- ¼ cup white wine
- 15 baby bella mushrooms
- 1 cup heavy cream
- 2 tbsp parsley, chopped

Directions

Total Time: approx. 40 minutes

1. Add butter and olive oil in a saucepan and heat over medium heat.
2. Season the chicken with salt and pepper, and brown on all sides for 6 minutes.
3. Put on a plate.
4. In a bowl, stir the onion soup mix with chicken broth and white wine, and add to the saucepan.
5. Simmer for 3 minutes and add the mushrooms and chicken.

6. Cover and simmer for another 20 minutes.

7. Stir in heavy cream and cook on low heat for 3 minutes.

8. Garnish with parsley.

Per serving:

- Cal 432
- Fat 35g
- Net Carbs 3.2g
- Protein 24g

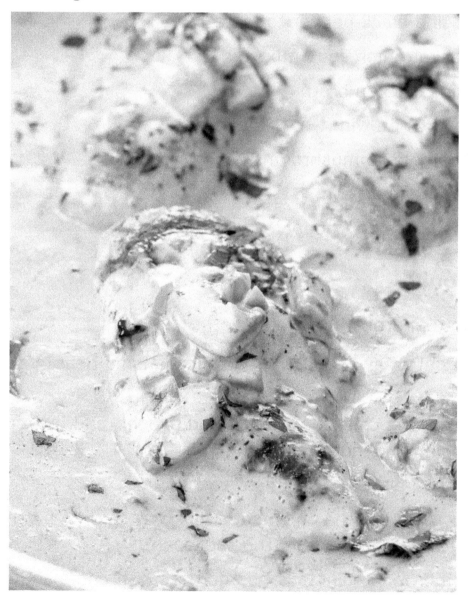

18. BACON ROLLED CHICKEN BREASTS

Ingredients

For 4 servings

- 1 green onion, chopped
- 1 cup gorgonzola cheese
- 1 lb chicken breasts, halved
- 4 oz bacon, sliced
- 2 tomatoes, chopped
- Salt and black pepper, to taste

Directions

Total Time: approx. 45 minutes

1. Preheat oven to 380 F.
2. Flatten the chicken breasts with a a rolling pin.
3. In a bowl, stir together the gorgonzola cheese, green onion, tomatoes, black pepper, and salt.
4. Spread the mixture on the chicken breasts.
5. Roll them up, and wrap each in a bacon slice.
6. Place the wrapped chicken breasts in a greased baking dish and roast in the oven for 30 minutes.
7. Serve.

Per serving:

- Cal 587

- Fat 43g
- Net Carbs 4.5g
- Protein 35g

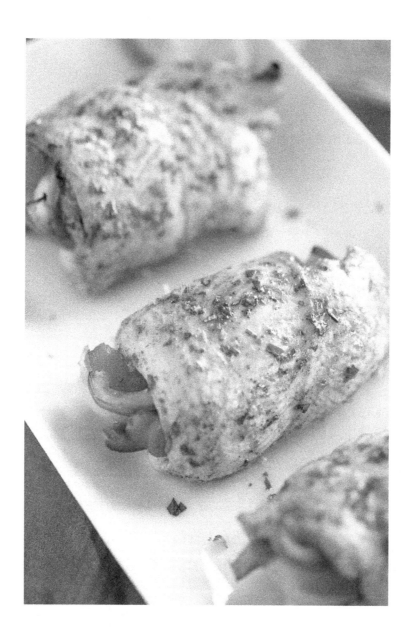

19. BAKED CHICKEN WRAPPED IN SMOKED BACON

Ingredients

For 2 servings

- 1 lb chicken breasts, flatten
- 1 tbsp olive oil
- 1 tbsp fresh parsley, chopped
- 1 tsp garlic paste, chopped
- ½ tsp sage
- Salt and black pepper, to taste
- ½ tsp smoked paprika
- 1 oz smoked bacon, sliced

Directions

Total Time: approx. 40 minutes

1. Mix garlic paste, sage, smoked paprika, salt, and black pepper in a small bowl; rub onto chicken and roll fillets in the smoked bacon slices.

2. Arrange on a greased with the olive oil baking dish and bake for 30 minutes at 390 F.

3. Plate the chicken and serve sprinkled with fresh parsley.

Per serving:

- Cal 556
- Fat 38g

- Net Carbs 2.3g
- Protein 51g

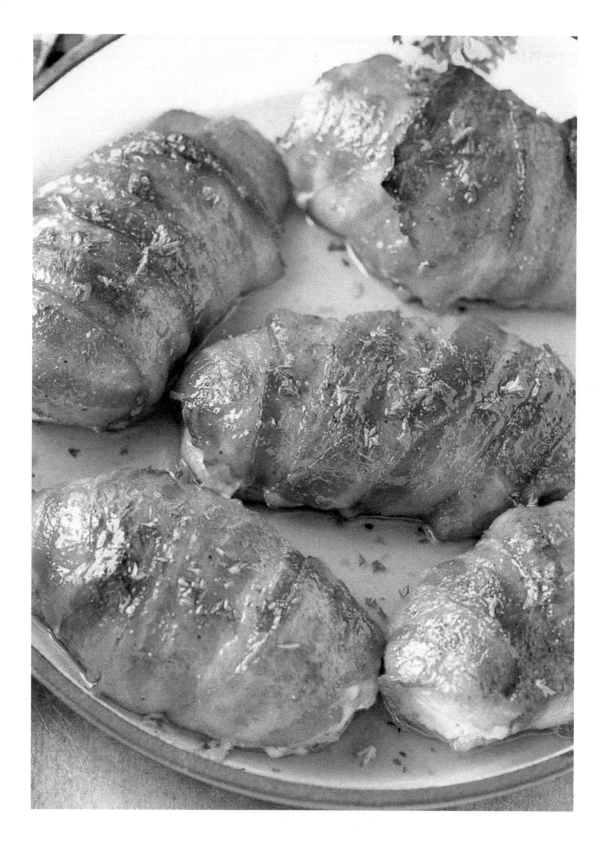

20. CHICKEN & CAULI RICE COLLARD GREEN ROLLS

Ingredients

For 4 servings

- 1 ½ lb chicken breasts, cubed
- 8 collard leaves
- 2 tbsp avocado oil
- 1 large yellow onion, chopped
- 2 garlic cloves, minced
- 1 jalapeño pepper, chopped
- 1 cup cauliflower rice
- 2 tsp hot sauce
- ¼ cup half-and-half
- Salt and black pepper to taste

Directions

Total Time: approx. 25 minutes

1. Warm avocado oil in a deep skillet and sauté onion and garlic until softened, 3 minutes.
2. Stir in jalapeño pepper, salt, and pepper.
3. Mix in chicken and cook until no longer pink on all sides, 10 minutes.
4. Add in cauliflower rice and hot sauce.
5. Sauté until the cauliflower slightly softens, 3 minutes.

6. Lay out the collards on a clean flat surface and spoon the curried mixture onto the middle part of the leaves, about 3 tbsp per leaf.

7. Spoon half-and-half on top, wrap the leaves, and serve immediately.

Per serving:

- Cal 441
- Net Carbs 1.8g
- Fat 32g
- Protein 41g

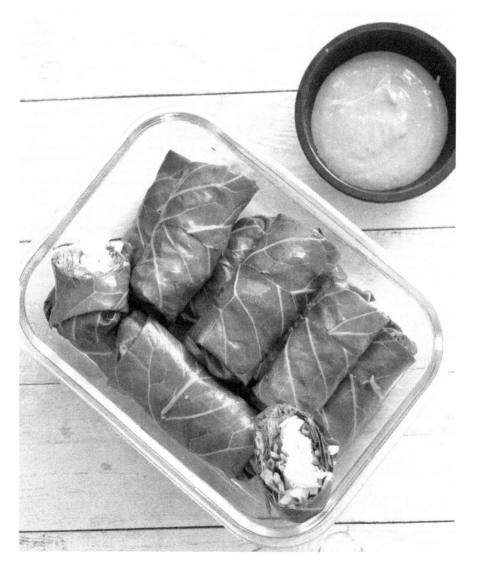

21. PESTO CHICKEN CACCIATORE

Ingredients

For 4 servings

- 2 lb chicken breasts, cubed
- 3 tbsp butter
- ½ lemon, juiced
- 3 tbsp basil pesto
- ¾ cup heavy cream
- ½ cup cream cheese, softened
- 1 celery, chopped
- ¼ cup chopped tomatoes
- 1 lb radishes, sliced
- ½ cup shredded Pepper Jack

Directions

Total Time: approx. 50 minutes

1. Preheat oven to 400 F.
2. In a bowl, combine lemon juice, pesto, heavy cream, and cream cheese; set aside.
3. Melt butter in a skillet and cook the chicken until no longer pink, 8 minutes.
4. Transfer to a greased casserole and spread the pesto mixture on top.
5. Top with celery, tomatoes, and radishes.
6. Sprinkle Pepper Jack cheese on top. Bake for 30 minutes or until the cheese melts and golden brown on top.

7. Serve warm and enjoy!

Per serving:

- Cal 671
- Net Carbs 0.8g
- Fat 47g
- Protein 49g

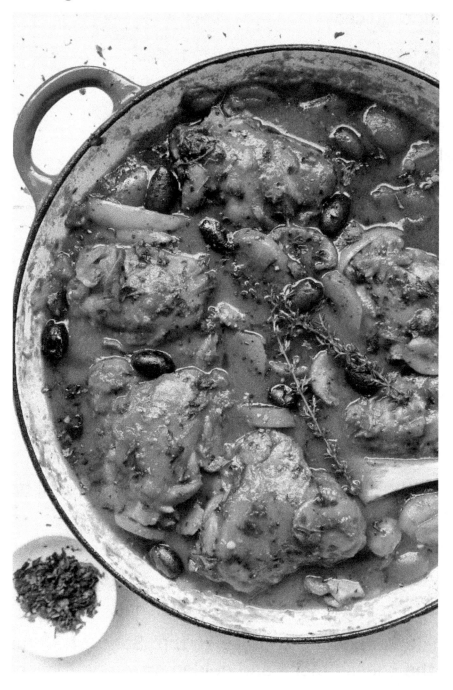

BEEF & LAMB

22. SKIRT STEAK WITH CAULI RICE & GREEN BEANS

Ingredients

For 4 servings

- Hot sauce (sugar- free) for topping
- 3 cups green beans, chopped
- 2 cups cauli rice
- 2 tbsp ghee
- 1 tbsp olive oil
- 1 lb skirt steak
- Salt and black pepper to taste
- 4 fresh eggs

Directions

Total Time: approx. 20 minutes

1. Put the cauli rice and green beans in a bowl. Sprinkle with a little water, and steam in the microwave for 90 seconds to be tender. Share into bowls.

2. Warm the ghee and olive oil in a skillet, season the beef with salt and black pepper, and brown for 5 minutes on each side.

3. Use a perforated spoon to scoop the meat onto the vegetables.

4. Wipe out the skillet and return to medium heat.

5. Crack in an egg, season with salt and pepper, and cook until the egg white has set, but the yolk is still runny 3 minutes.

6. Remove egg onto the vegetable bowl and fry the remaining 3 eggs.

7. Add to the other bowls. Drizzle with hot sauce and serve.

Per serving:

- Cal 334

- Fat 25g

- Net Carbs 6.3g

- Protein 14g

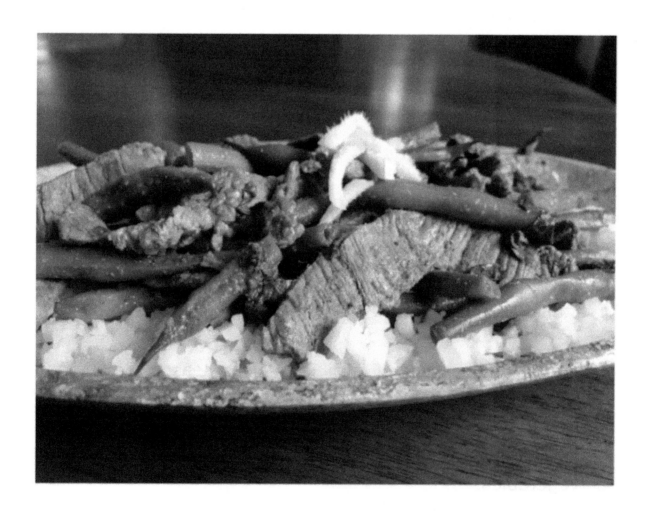

23. TRADITIONAL SCOTTISH BEEF WITH PARSNIPS

Ingredients

For 4 servings

- 2 tbsp olive oil
- 12 oz canned corn beef, cubed
- 1 onion, chopped
- 4 parsnips, chopped
- 1 carrot, chopped
- 1 garlic clove, minced
- Salt and black pepper to taste
- 1 cup vegetable broth 2 tsp rosemary leaves
- 1 tbsp Worcestershire sauce
- ½ small cabbage, shredded

Directions

Total Time: approx. 45 minutes

1. Add the onion, garlic, carrots, rosemary, and parsnips to a warm olive oil over medium heat.
2. Stir and cook for a minute. Pour in the vegetable broth and Worcestershire sauce.
3. Stir the mixture and cook the ingredients on low heat for 25 minutes.
4. Stir in the cabbage and corn beef, season with salt and pepper, and cook for 10 minutes.

Per serving:

- Cal 321
- Fat 16g
- Net Carbs 2.3g
- Protein 13g

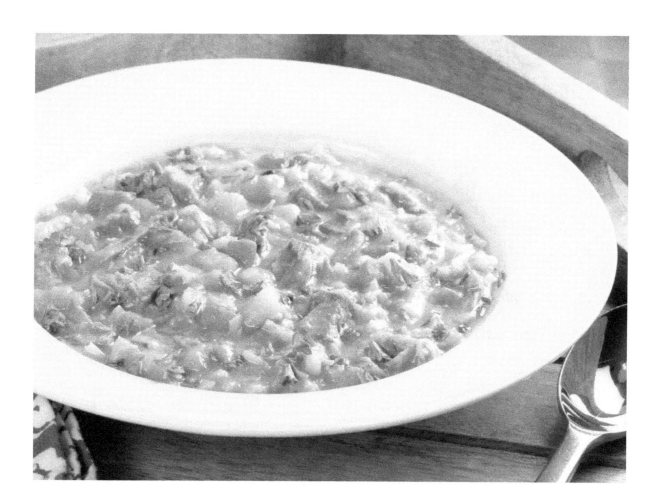

24. SUNDAY BEEF GRATIN

Ingredients

For 4 servings

- 1 tbsp olive oil
- 1 onion, chopped
- 1 lb ground beef
- 2 garlic cloves, minced
- Salt and black pepper to taste
- 1 cup mozzarella, shredded
- 1 cup fontina cheese, shredded
- 14 oz canned tomatoes, diced
- 2 tbsp sesame seeds, toasted
- 20 dill pickle slices

Directions

Total Time: approx. 35 minutes

1. Preheat the oven to 390 F.
2. Heat olive oil in a pan over medium heat, place in the beef, garlic, salt, onion, and black pepper, and cook for 5 minutes.
3. Remove and set to a baking dish, stir in half of the tomatoes and mozzarella cheese.
4. Lay the pickle slices on top, spread over the fontina cheese and sesame seeds, and place in the oven to bake for 20 minutes.

Per serving:

- Cal 523
- Fat 43g
- Net Carbs 6.5g
- Protein 36g

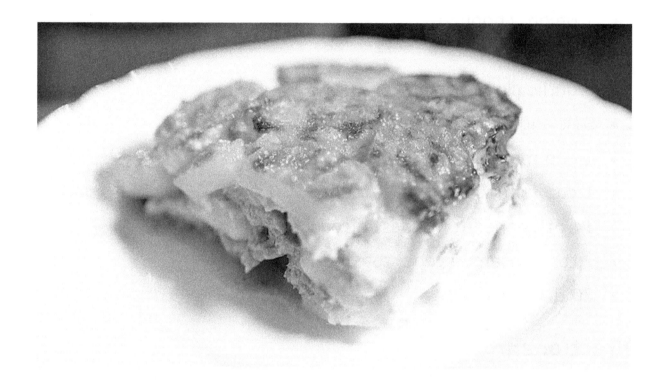

25. BEEF BURGERS WITH LETTUCE & AVOCADO

Ingredients

For 2 servings

- ½ lb ground beef
- 1 green onion, chopped
- ½ tsp garlic powder
- 1 tbsp butter
- Salt and black pepper to taste
- 1 tbsp olive oil
- ½ tsp Dijon mustard
- 1 low carb buns, halved
- 2 tbsp mayonnaise
- ½ tsp balsamic vinegar
- 2 tbsp iceberg lettuce, torn
- 1 avocado, sliced

Directions

Total Time: approx. 15 minutes

1. In a bowl, mix ground beef, green onion, garlic powder, mustard, salt, and pepper; create 2 burgers.

2. Heat the butter and olive oil in a skillet and cook the burgers for 3 minutes per side.

3. Fill the buns with lettuce, mayonnaise, balsamic vinegar, burgers, and avocado slices to serve.

Per serving:

- Cal 778
- Fat 62g
- Net Carbs 5.6g
- Protein 34g

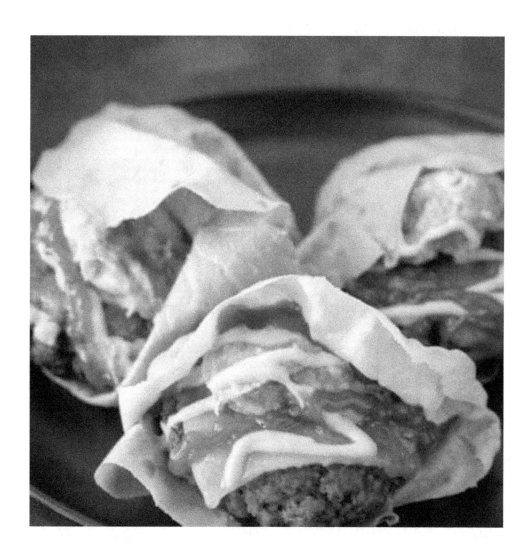

26. CABBAGE & BEEF STACKS

Ingredients

For 4 servings

- 1 lb chuck steak
- 1 headcanon cabbage, grated
- ¼ cup olive oil
- 3 tbsp coconut flour
- 1 tsp Italian mixed herb blend
- ½ cup bone broth

Directions

Total Time: approx. 55 minutes

1. Preheat the oven to 380 F.
2. Slice the steak thinly across the grain with a sharp knife.
3. In a zipper bag, add coconut flour and beef slices.
4. Seal the bag and shake to coat.
5. Make little mounds of cabbage in a greased baking dish.
6. Drizzle with some olive oil.
7. Remove the beef strips from the coconut flour mixture, shake off the excess flour, and place 2-3 beef strips on each cabbage mound.
8. Sprinkle the Italian herb blend and drizzle again with the remaining olive oil.
9. Roast for 30 minutes.
10. Remove the pan and carefully pour in the broth.

11. Return to the oven and roast further for 10 minutes, until beef cooks through.

12. Serve and enjoy!

Per serving:

- Cal 231
- Net Carbs 1.5g
- Fat 14g
- Protein 18g

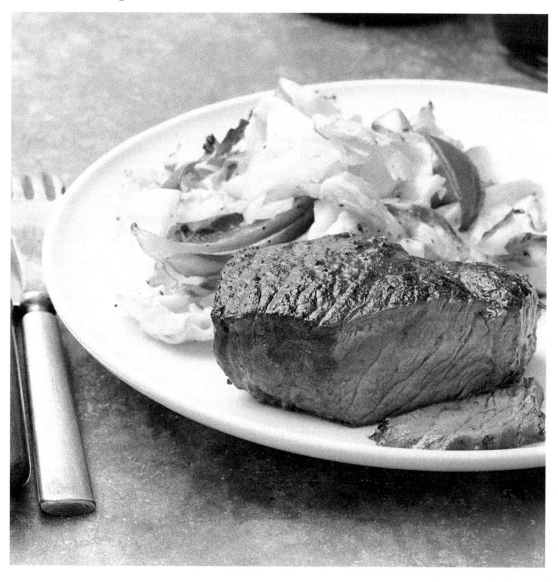

FISH & SEAFOOD

27. BAKED TROUT & ASPARAGUS FOIL PACKETS

Ingredients

For 2 servings

- ½ lb asparagus spears
- 1 tbsp garlic puree
- ½ lb deboned trout, butterflied
- Salt and black pepper to taste
- 1 sprigs rosemary
- 2 sprigs thyme
- 2 tbsp butter
- ½ medium red onion, sliced
- 2 lemon slices

Directions

Total Time: approx. 25 minutes

1. Preheat the oven to 400 F.
2. Rub the trout with garlic puree, salt, and pepper.
3. Prepare two aluminum foil squares.
4. Place the fish on each square.
5. Divide the asparagus and onion between the squares, top with a pinch of salt and pepper, a sprig of rosemary and thyme, and 1 tbsp of butter.
6. Also, lay the lemon slices on the fish.

7. Wrap and close the fish packets securely, and place them on a baking sheet.

8. Bake in the oven for 15 minutes.

9. Serve.

Per serving:

- Cal 498
- Fat 39g
- Net Carbs 4.6g
- Protein 27g

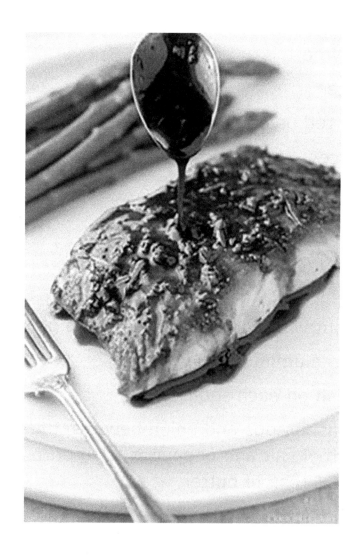

28. GREEN TUNA TRAYBAKE

Ingredients

For 4 servings

- 1 (15 oz) can tuna in water, drained and flaked
- 1 bunch asparagus, trimmed and cut into 1-inch pieces
- 1 cup green beans, chopped
- 1 tbsp butter
- 2 tbsp arrowroot starch
- 2 cups coconut milk
- 4 zucchinis, spiralized
- 1 cup grated Parmesan cheese

Directions

Total Time: approx. 40 minutes

1. Preheat the oven to 370 F.
2. Melt butter in a skillet and sauté the green beans and asparagus until softened, about 5 minutes; set aside.
3. In a saucepan over medium heat, mix arrowroot starch with coconut milk.
4. Bring to a boil and cook with frequent stirring until thickened, 3 minutes.
5. Stir in half of Parmesan cheese until melted.
6. Mix in the green beans, asparagus, zucchinis, and tuna.
7. Transfer the mixture to a baking dish and sprinkle with the remaining Parmesan cheese.
8. Bake until the cheese is melted and golden, 1820 minutes.
9. Serve.

Per serving:

- Cal 392
- Net Carbs 8g
- Fats 34g
- Protein 9g

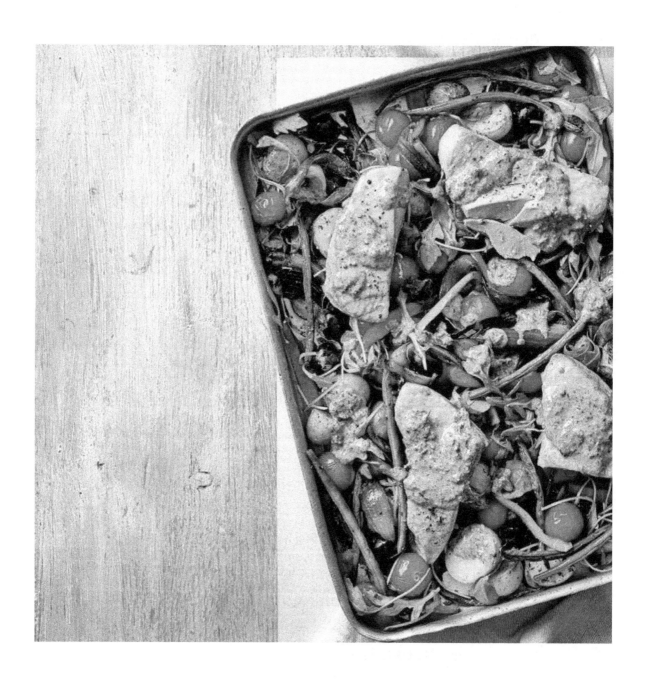

VEGETABLE SIDES & DAIRY

29. FETA & OLIVE PIZZA

Ingredients

- For 4 servings
- 1 tbsp olive oil
- ½ cup almond flour
- 1 tbsp ground psyllium husk
- ¼ tsp salt
- ¼ tsp red chili flakes
- ¼ tsp dried Greek seasoning
- 1 cup crumbled feta cheese
- 3 plum tomatoes, sliced
- 6 Kalamata olives, chopped
- 5 basil leaves, chopped

Directions

Total Time: approx. 30 minutes

1. Preheat oven to 390 F.
2. Line a baking sheet with parchment paper.
3. In a bowl, mix almond flour, salt, psyllium powder, olive oil, and 1 cup of lukewarm water until; stir until a dough forms.
4. Spread the mixture on the baking sheet and bake for 10 minutes.
5. Sprinkle the red chili flakes and Greek seasoning on the crust and top with the feta cheese.
6. Arrange the tomatoes and olives on top. Bake for 10 minutes.

7. Garnish the pizza with basil, slice, and serve warm.

Per serving:

- Cal 281
- Net Carbs 4.5g
- Fats 12g
- Protein 8g

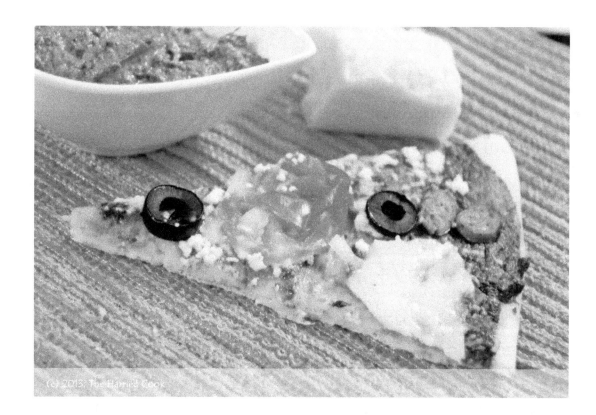

30. CHARGRILLED ZUCCHINI WITH AVOCADO PESTO

Ingredients

For 4 servings

- 1 avocado, chopped
- 3 oz spinach, chopped
- 2 zucchinis, sliced
- ¾ cup olive oil
- 2 tbsp melted butter
- 2 oz pecans
- 1 garlic clove, minced
- Juice of 1 lemon
- Salt and black pepper to taste

Directions

Total Time: approx. 20 minutes

1. Put the spinach in a food processor and avocado, lemon juice, garlic, olive oil, and pecans and blend until smooth; season with salt and pepper.

2. Pour the pesto into a bowl and set it aside.

3. Season zucchini with salt, pepper, and butter.

4. Preheat a grill pan over medium heat and cook the zucchini slices until browned, 8-10 minutes in total.

5. Remove to a plate, spoon the pesto to the side, and serve.

Per serving:

- Cal 548
- Net Carbs 6g
- Fat 46g
- Protein 25g

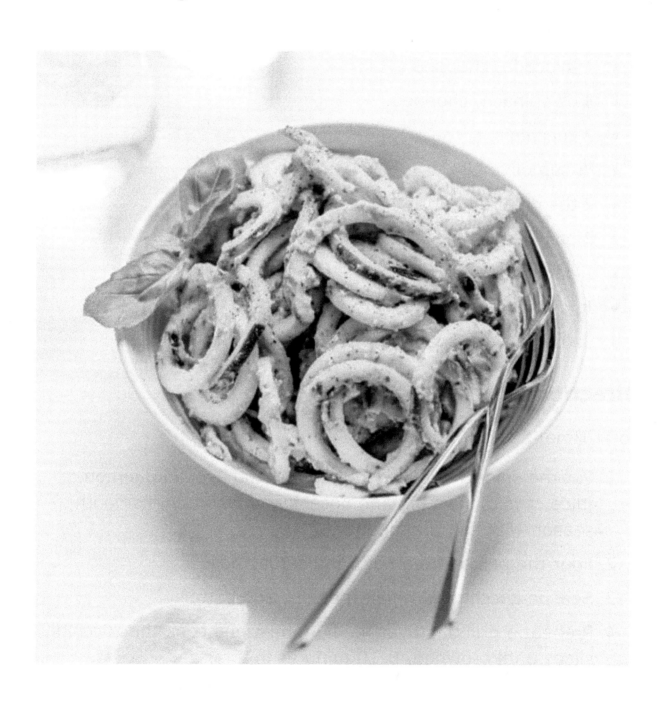

31. WALNUT & FETA LOAF

Ingredients

For 4 servings

- 1 green bell pepper, chopped
- 1 red bell pepper, chopped
- 2 white onions, chopped
- 4 garlic cloves, minced
- 1 lb feta, cubed
- 3 tbsp olive oil
- 2 tbsp soy sauce
- ¾ cup chopped walnuts
- Salt and black pepper
- 1 tbsp Italian mixed herbs
- ½ tsp Swerve sugar
- ¼ cup golden flaxseed meal
- 1 tbsp sesame seeds ½ cup tomato sauce

Directions

Total Time: approx. 60 minutes

1. Preheat oven to 350 F.

2. In a bowl, combine olive oil, onions, garlic, feta, soy sauce, walnuts, salt, pepper, Italian herbs, Swerve, and flaxseed meal and mix with your hands.

3. Pour the mixture into a bowl and stir in sesame seeds and bell peppers.

4. Transfer the mixture into a greased loaf and spoon tomato sauce on top.

5. Bake for 45 minutes.

6. Turn onto a chopping board, slice, and serve.

Per serving:

- Cal 429
- Net Carbs 2.5g
- Fat 28g
- Protein 24g

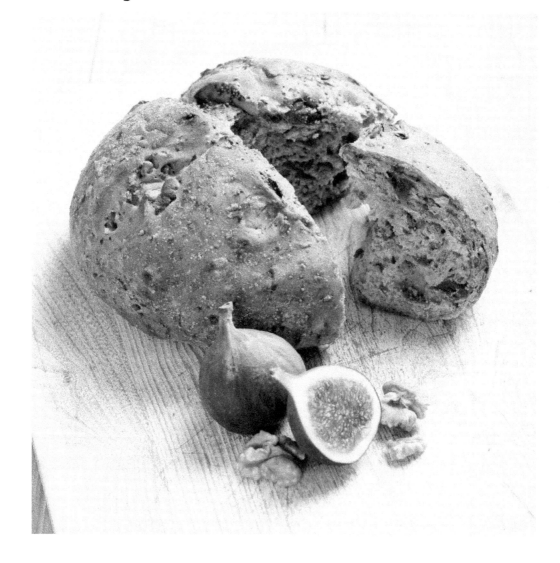

VEGAN

32. STEAMED BOK CHOY WITH THYME & GARLIC

Ingredients

For 4 servings

- 2 lb Bok choy, sliced
- 2 tbsp coconut oil
- 2 tbsp soy sauce, sugar- free
- 1 tsp garlic, minced
- ½ tsp thyme, chopped
- ½ tsp red pepper flakes
- Salt and black pepper to taste

Directions

Total Time: approx. 15 minutes

1. Place a pan over medium heat and warm the coconut oil.
2. Add in garlic and cook until soft, 1 minute.
3. Stir in the bok choy, red pepper, soy sauce, black pepper, salt, and thyme and cook until everything is heated through, about 5 minutes.
4. Serve.

Per serving:

- Cal 132
- Fat 9.5g
- Net Carbs 3.5g
- Protein 4.9g

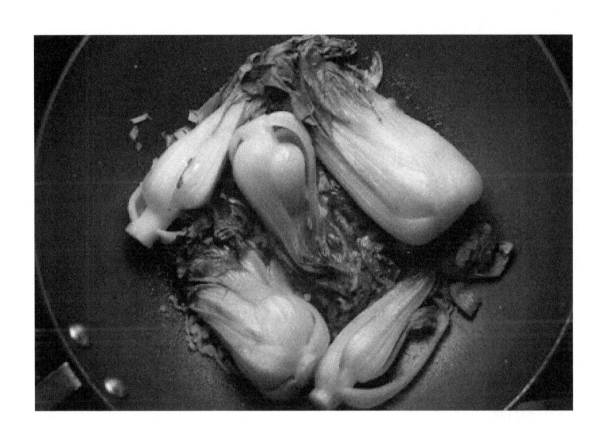

33. STICKY TOFU WITH CUCUMBER & TOMATO SALAD

Ingredients

For 4 servings

- 2 tbsp olive oil
- 12 oz tofu, sliced
- 1 cup green onions, chopped
- 1 garlic clove, minced
- 2 tbsp vinegar
- 1 tbsp sriracha sauc e Salad
- 1 tbsp fresh lemon juice
- 2 tbsp extra virgin olive oil
- Salt and black pepper to taste
- 1 tsp fresh dill weed
- 1 cucumber, sliced
- 2 tomatoes, sliced

Directions

Total Time: approx. 15 min + chilling time

1. Put tofu slices, garlic, sriracha sauce, vinegar, and green onions in a bowl; allow to settle for approximately 30 minutes.
2. Warm the olive oil in a skillet over medium heat.
3. Cook tofu for 5 minutes until golden brown.

4. In a salad plate, arrange tomatoes and cucumber slices, season with salt and pepper, drizzle lemon juice and extra virgin olive oil, and scatter dill all over.

5. Top with the tofu and serve.

Per serving:

- Cal 371
- Fat 31g
- Net Carbs 7.7g
- Protein 17g

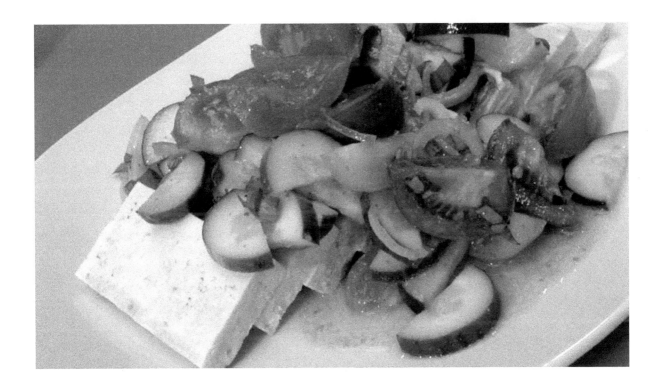

SNACKS & APPETIZERS

34. FLAXSEED TOASTS WITH AVOCADO PATÉ

Ingredients

For 4 servings

- 1 pinch of salt
- ½ cup flaxseed meal

For the avocado paté

- 3 ripe avocados, chopped
- 4 tbsp Greek yogurt
- 2 tbsp chopped green onions
- 1 lemon, zested and juiced
- Black pepper to taste
- Smoked paprika to garnish

Directions

Total Time: approx. 25 minutes

1. Preheat oven to 350 F.
2. Place a skillet over medium heat.
3. Put in flaxseed meal, ¼ cup water, and salt and mix continually to form the dough into a ball.
4. Place the dough between 2 parchment papers, place on a flat surface, and flatten thinly with a rolling pin.
5. Remove the papers and cut the pastry into tortilla chips.
6. Place on a baking sheet and bake for 8-12 minutes or until crispy.

7. In a bowl, mix avocados, yogurt, green onions, lemon zest and juice, and black pepper until evenly combined.

8. Spread the paté on the toasts and garnish with paprika. Serve immediately.

Per serving:

- Cal 359
- Net Carbs 4g
- Fat 31g
- Protein 7g

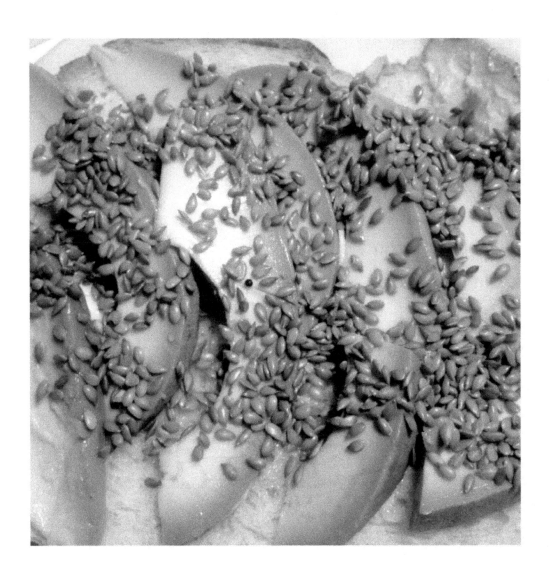

35. CARAMELIZED ONION & CREAM CHEESE SPREAD

Ingredients

For 4 servings

- 2 cups sour cream
- 8 oz cream cheese, softened
- ½ tbsp Worcestershire sauce
- 2 tbsp butter
- 3 yellow onions, thinly sliced
- 1 tsp Swerve sugar
- ¼ cup white wine
- Salt to taste

Directions

Total Time: approx. 35 minutes

1. Melt the butter in a skillet over medium heat.
2. Add in the onions, Swerve sugar, and salt.
3. Cook with frequent stirring for 10-15 minutes.
4. Add in white wine, stir, and allow sizzling out, 10 minutes.
5. In a serving bowl, mix sour cream and cream cheese.
6. Add in caramelized onions and Worcestershire sauce and stir well into the cream.
7. Serve with celery sticks if desired.

Per serving:

- Cal 379
- Net Carbs 8g
- Fat 34g
- Protein 8g

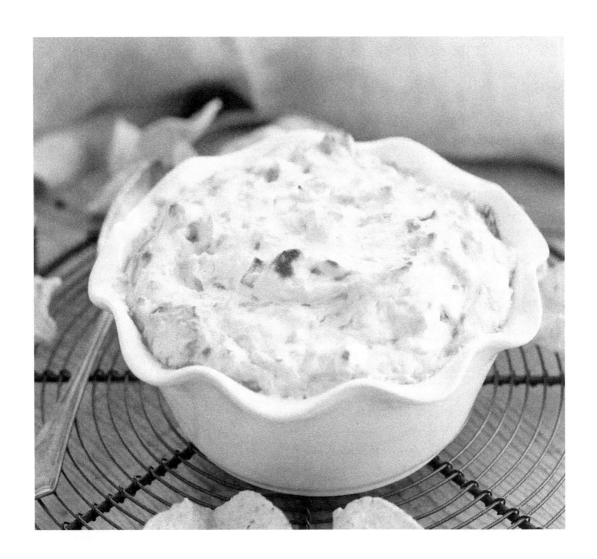

36. MAPLE TAHINI STRAWS

Ingredients

For 4 servings

For the puff pastry

- 3 tbsp coconut flour
- ¼ cup almond flour
- ½ tsp xanthan gum
- 3 whole eggs
- 4 tbsp cream cheese, softened
- ¼ teaspoon cream of tartar
- ¼ cup butter, cold
- 3 tbsp erythritol
- 1 tsp vanilla extract
- ½ tsp salt

For the filling

- 1 tbsp sugar- free maple syrup
- 2 tbsp poppy seeds
- 2 tbsp sesame seeds
- 1 egg, beaten
- 3 tbsp tahini

Directions

Total Time: approx. 30 min + cooling time

1. Preheat oven to 350 F.
2. Line a baking tray with parchment paper.
3. In a bowl, mix almond and coconut flours, xanthan gum, and salt.
4. Add in cream cheese, cream of tartar, and butter; mix with an electric mixer until crumbly.
5. Add erythritol and vanilla extract until mixed.
6. Then, pour in 3 eggs one after another while mixing until formed into a ball.
7. Flatten the dough on a clean flat surface, cover with plastic wrap, and refrigerate for 1 hour.

8. Dust a clean flat surface with almond flour, unwrap the dough, and roll out the dough into a large rectangle.
9. In a bowl, mix maple syrup and tahini and spread the mixture over the pastry.
10. Sprinkle with half of the sesame seeds and cut the dough into 16 strips.
11. Fold each strip in half. Brush the top with the beaten egg, sprinkle with the remaining seeds and poppy seeds.
12. Twist the pastry three to four times into straws and place on the baking sheet.
13. Bake until golden brown, 15 minutes. Serve with chocolate sauce.

Per serving:

- Cal 351
- Net Carbs 3.1g
- Fat 31g
- Protein 11 g

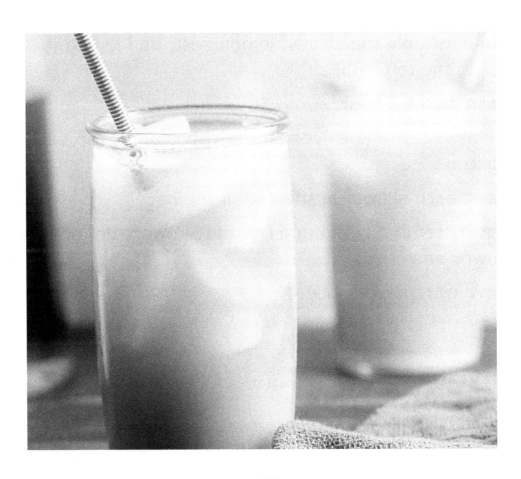

37. BACON & TOFU POPS

Ingredients

For 4 servings

- 2 tbsp butter
- 12 slices bacon
- 1 (14 oz) block tofu, cubed
- 2 tbsp chives, chopped
- 1 lemon, zested and juiced
- 12 mini skewers

Directions

Total Time: approx. 20 min + chilling time

1. In a bowl, mix the chives, lemon zest, and lemon juice and toss in the tofu cubes.
2. Marinate for 1 hour.
3. Take the zest and chives off the cubes and wrap each tofu in a bacon slice.
4. Insert each skewer at the end of the bacon.
5. Melt butter in a skillet and fry tofu skewers until the bacon browns and crisps.
6. Serve with mayo sauce.

Per serving:

- Cal 389
- Net Carbs 9g

- Fat 22g
- Protein 18g

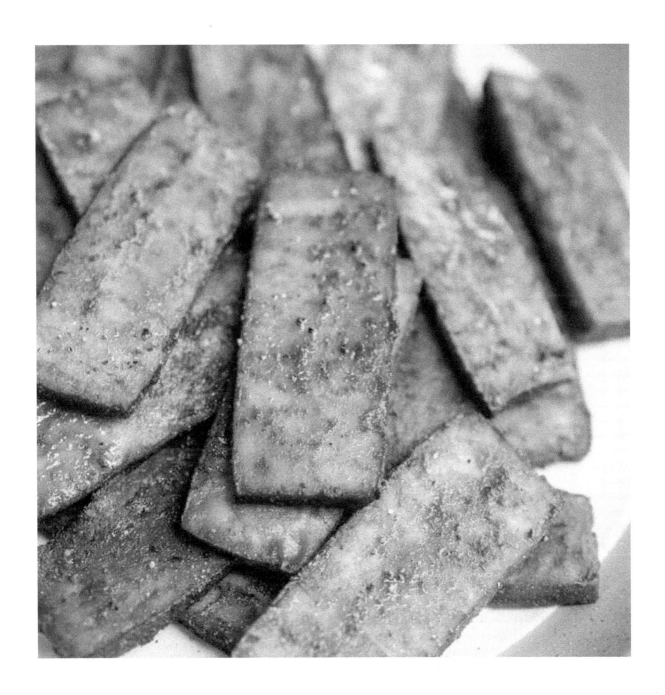

38. ROSEMARY FETA CHEESE BOMBS

Ingredients

For 4 servings

- 6 tbsp butter
- 2 /3 cup almond flour
- 3 eggs
- 1 cup crumbled feta cheese
- ½ cup heavy whipping cream
- 1 tbsp olive oil
- 2 sprigs rosemary
- 2 white onions, thinly sliced
- 2 tbsp red wine vinegar
- 1 tsp Swerve brown sugar

Directions

Total Time: approx. 50 minutes

1. Preheat oven to 350 F.
2. Line a baking tray with parchment paper.
3. In a saucepan, warm 1 cup of water and butter.
4. Bring to a boil and add in almond flour, beating vigorously until ball forms.
5. Turn the heat off; keep beating while adding the eggs, one at a time, until the dough is smooth and slightly thickened.
6. Scoop mounds of the dough onto the baking dish.
7. Press a hole in the center of each mound.
8. Bake for 20 minutes until risen and golden.
9. Remove from the oven and pierce the sides of the buns with a toothpick.
10. Return to oven and bake for 2 minutes until crispy. Set aside to cool.

11. Tear out the middle part of the bun (keep the torn out part) to create a hole in the bun for the cream filling.
12. Set aside. Heat olive oil in a saucepan and sauté onions and rosemary for 2 minutes.
13. Stir in Swerve sugar and vinegar and cook to bubble for 3 minutes or until caramelized.
14. In a bowl, beat whipping cream and feta together. Spoon the mixture into a piping bag and press a spoonful of the mixture into the buns.
15. Cover with the torn out portion of pastry and top with onion relish to serve.

Per serving:

- Cal 379
- Net Carbs 2.5g
- Fat 37g
- Protein 10g

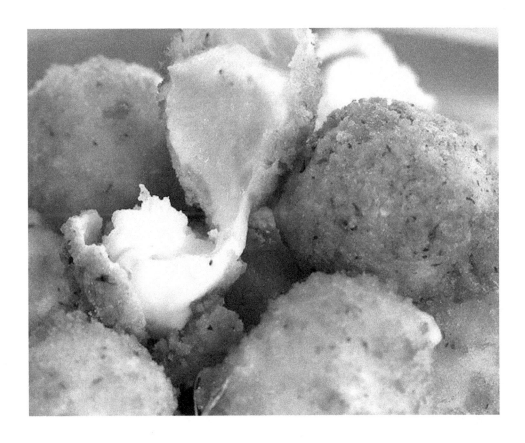

39. MUSHROOM & FETA SKEWERS

Ingredients

For 2 servings

- ½ lb white button mushrooms, quartered
- 14 oz block feta cheese, cubed
- 2 tbsp olive oil
- 2 red onions, cut into wedges
- 1 tsp Chinese five-spice
- 1 lemon, juiced
- 2 tbsp chopped parsley

Directions

Total Time: approx. 20 minutes

1. Thread feta, mushrooms, and onions alternately on the skewers.
2. In a bowl, mix olive oil, Chinese five-spice, and lemon juice.
3. Brush the skewers with the mixture.
4. Cook in a grill pan over high heat until the vegetables lightly char, about 10 minutes.
5. Garnish with parsley and serve.

Per serving:

- Cal 368
- Net Carbs 6.9g
- Fat 27g

- Protein 25g

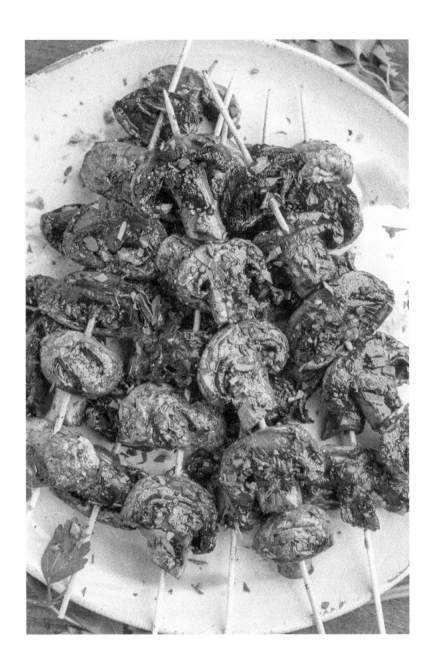

SMOOTHIES
&
BEVERAGES

40. GREEN SMOOTHIE

Ingredients

For 4 servings

- ¼ cup cold almond milk
- 1 tbsp cold heavy cream
- 4 avocados, halved and pitted
- 4 tbsp Swerve sugar
- 1 tsp vanilla extract

Directions

Total Time: approx. 5 minutes

1. In a blender, add avocado, swerve sugar, milk, vanilla extract, and heavy cream.
2. Process until smooth. Pour the mixture into 2 glasses and serve.

Per serving:

- Cal 390
- Net Carbs 2g
- Fat 29g
- Protein 6.9g

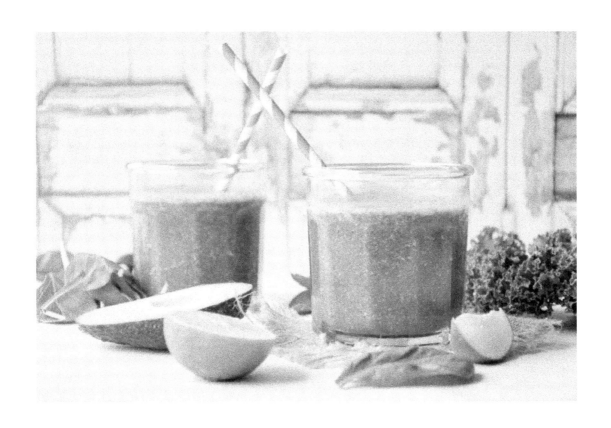

SWEETS & DESSERTS

41. MASCARPONE CREAM MOUSSE

Ingredients

For 6 servings

For the mascarpone

- 8 oz heavy cream
- 8 oz mascarpone cheese
- 4 tbsp cocoa powder 4 tbsp xylitol

For the vanilla mousse

- 3.5 oz heavy cream
- 3.5 oz cream cheese
- 1 tsp vanilla extract
- 2 tbsp xylitol

Directions

Total Time: approx. 15 minutes

1. Beat mascarpone cheese, heavy cream, cocoa powder, and xylitol with an electric mixer until creamy.

2. Do not over mix, however. In another bowl, whisk all the mousse ingredients until smooth.

3. Gradually fold vanilla mousse mixture into the mascarpone one until well incorporated.

4. Spoon into dessert cups and serve.

Per serving:

- Cal 409
- Net Carbs 5.9g
- Fat 32g
- Protein 7.9g

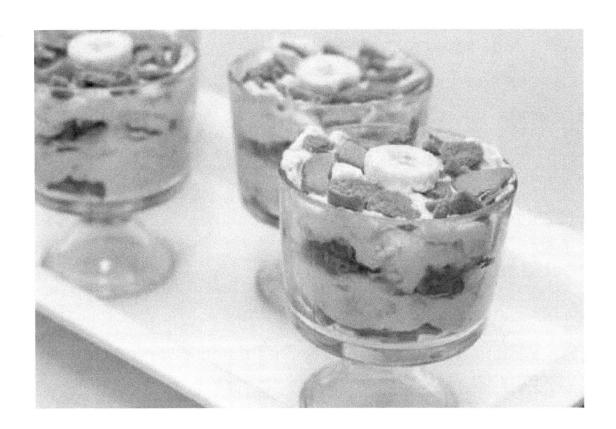

42. MOJITO MOUSSE WITH BLACKBERRIES

Ingredients

For 4 servings

- ½ cup Swerve confectioner's sugar
- 2 ½ cups sour cream
- 3 cups heavy cream
- 3 limes, juiced
- ½ tsp vanilla extract
- Chopped mint to garnish
- 12 blackberries for topping

Directions

Total Time: approx. 10 min + chilling time

1. In a stand mixer, beat heavy cream and Swerve sugar until creamy.
2. Add sour cream, lime juice, and vanilla; combine smoothly.
3. Divide between 4 dessert cups, cover with plastic wrap, and refrigerate for 2 hours.
4. Remove, garnish with mint leaves, top with blackberries, and serve.

Per serving:

- Cal 489
- Net Carbs 8.7g
- Fat 43g

- Protein 3.9g

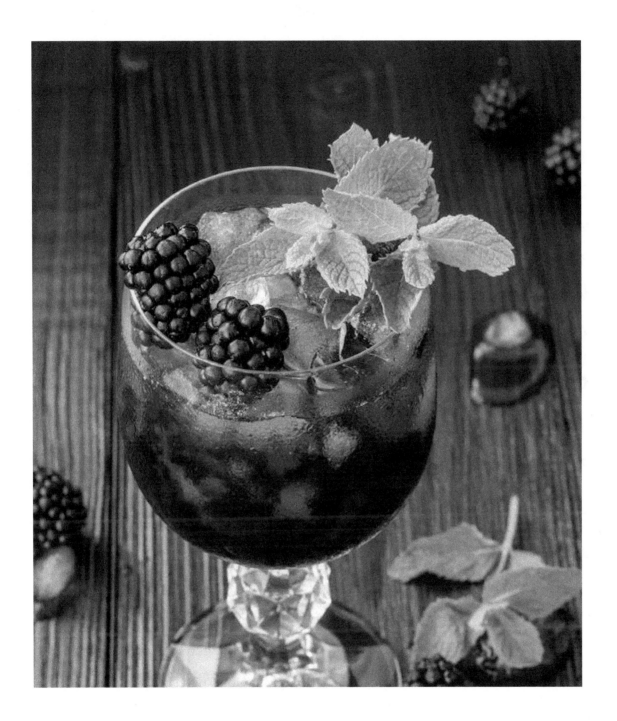

43. SPEEDY CHOCOLATE PEPPERMINT MOUSSE

Ingredients

For 4 servings

- 4 oz cream cheese
- 1 /3 cup coconut cream
- ¼ cup Swerve sugar, divided
- 3 tbsp cocoa powder
- ¾ tsp peppermint extract
- ½ tsp vanilla extract

Directions

Total Time: approx. 10 min + chilling time

1. Place 2 tbsp of Swerve, cream cheese, and cocoa powder in a blender.
2. Add in peppermint extract and ¼ cup warm water; process until smooth.
3. In a bowl, whip vanilla extract, coconut cream, and remaining Swerve using a whisk.
4. Fetch out 5 tbsp for garnishing.
5. Fold in cocoa mixture until thoroughly combined.
6. Spoon the mousse into cups and refrigerate.
7. Garnish with whipped cream.

Per serving:

- Cal 169

- Net Carbs 2g
- Fat 15.9g
- Protein 2.9g

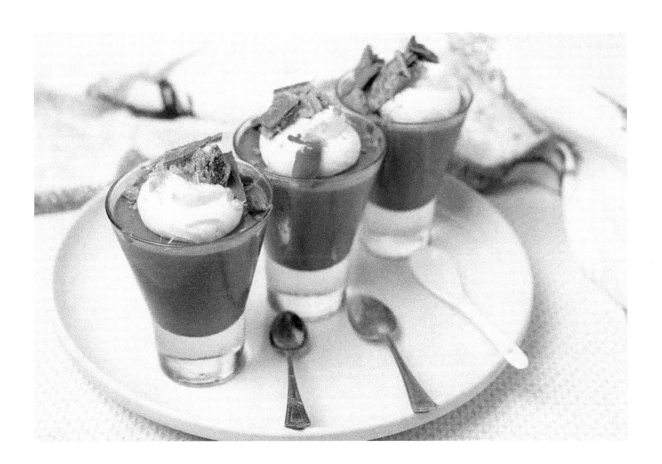

44. STRAWBERRY CHOCOLATE MOUSSE

Ingredients

For 2 servings

- 3 eggs
- ½ cup dark chocolate chips
- 1 cup heavy cream
- 1 cup fresh strawberries, sliced

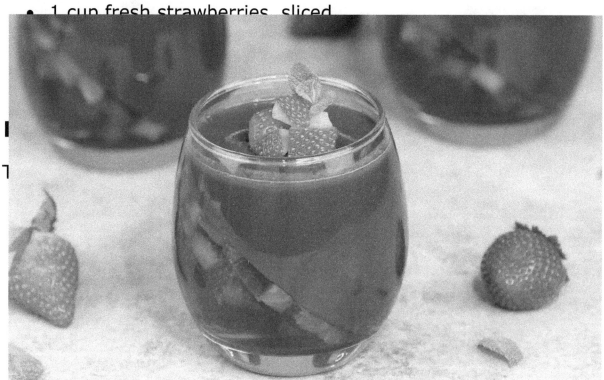

slices, and chill in the fridge for at least 30 minutes before serving.

Per serving:

- Cal 567
- Fat 46g
- Net Carbs 9.6g
- Protein 14g

45. FLUFFY LEMON CURD MOUSSE WITH WALNUTS

Ingredients

For 4 servings

For the mousse

- 1 cup cold heavy cream
- 8 oz cream cheese
- ¼ cup Swerve sugar
- 1 tsp vanilla extract ½ lemon, juiced

For the caramel nuts

- 1 cup walnuts, chopped
- 2 /3 cup Swerve brown sugar
- A pinch salt

Directions

Total Time: approx. 20 min + chilling time

1. In a stand mixer, beat cream cheese and heavy cream until you get a creamy consistency. Add vanilla, Swerve sugar, and lemon juice until smooth. Divide the mixture between 4 dessert cups. Cover with plastic wrap and refrigerate for at least 2 hours. *For the caramel walnuts:*

2. Add Swerve sugar to a large skillet and cook over medium heat with frequent stirring until melted and golden brown. Mix in 2 tbsp of water and salt and cook further until syrupy and slightly thickened.

3. Turn the heat off and quickly mix in the walnuts until well coated in the caramel; let sit for 5 minutes. Remove the mousse from the fridge and top with the caramel walnuts. Serve immediately.

Per serving:

- Cal 521
- Net Carbs 8g
- Fat 53g
- Protein 7g

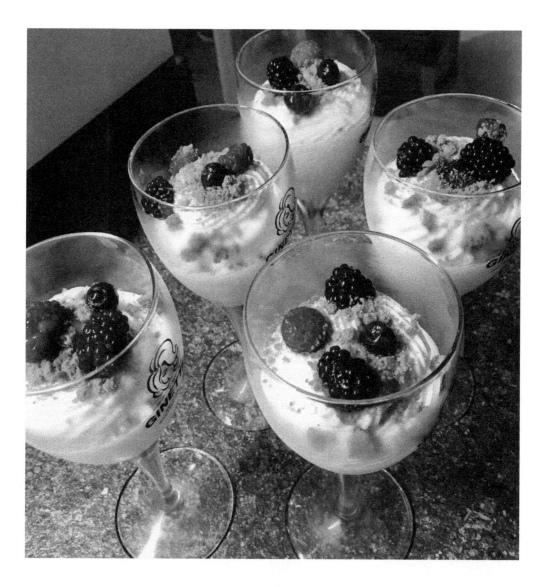

46. CHOCOLATE ALMOND ICE CREAM TREATS

Ingredients

For 4 servings

Ice cream

- ½ cup heavy whipping cream
- ½ tsp vanilla extract
- ½ tsp xanthan gum
- ¼ cup almond butter
- ½ cup half and half
- cup almond milk
- ¼ tsp stevia powder
- ½ tbsp vegetable glycerin
- tbsp erythritol **Chocolate**
- ¼ cup cocoa butter pieces, chopped
- ½ tsp THM super sweet blend
- ¾ cup coconut oil
- 2 oz unsweetened chocolate

Directions

Total Time: approx. 20 min + cooling time

1. In a bowl, blend all ice cream ingredients until smooth.
2. Place in an ice cream maker and follow the instructions. Spread the ice cream into a lined pan and freezer for about 4 hours.

3. Mix all chocolate ingredients in a microwave-safe bowl and heat until melted.

4. Allow cooling. Remove ice cream from the freezer and slice into bars.

5. Dip into the cooled chocolate mixture and return to the freezer for about 10 minutes before serving.

Per serving:

- Cal 305
- Fat 25g
- Net Carbs 5.3g
- Protein 6.2g

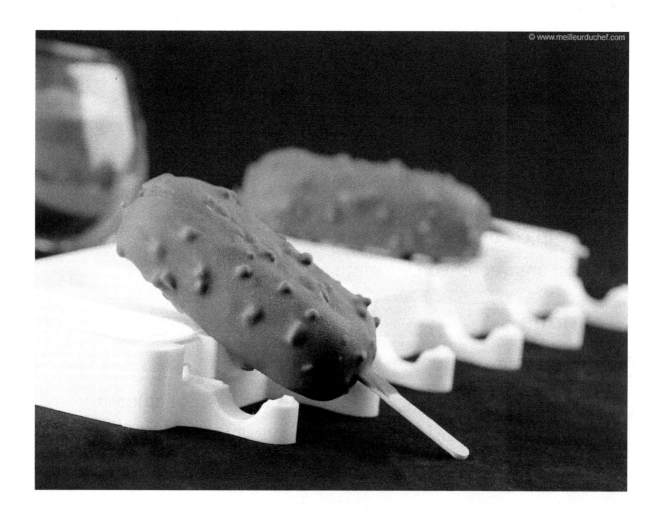

47. CHOCOLATE MOCHA MOUSSE CUPS

Ingredients

For 4 servings

- 2 tbsp butter, softened
- 8 oz cream cheese, softened
- 2 /3 cup heavy whipping cream
- 3 tbsp sour cream
- 1 /3 cup erythritol
- 3 tsp instant coffee powder
- ¼ cup cocoa powder
- 1 ½ tsp Swerve sugar
- ½ tsp vanilla extract

Directions

Total Time: approx. 10 minutes

1. Beat cream cheese, sour cream, and butter with an electric hand mixer until smooth.
2. Add in vanilla, erythritol, coffee and cocoa powders and mix thoroughly until all ingredients are well incorporated.
3. In a separate bowl, beat whipping cream and Swerve sugar until soft peaks form.
4. Fold 1/3 of the whipped cream mixture into the cream cheese mixture to lighten a bit.
5. Stir in the remaining mixture until well incorporated.
6. Spoon into dessert cups. Serve.

Per serving:

- Cal 310
- Net Carbs 4g
- Fat 29g
- Protein 5g

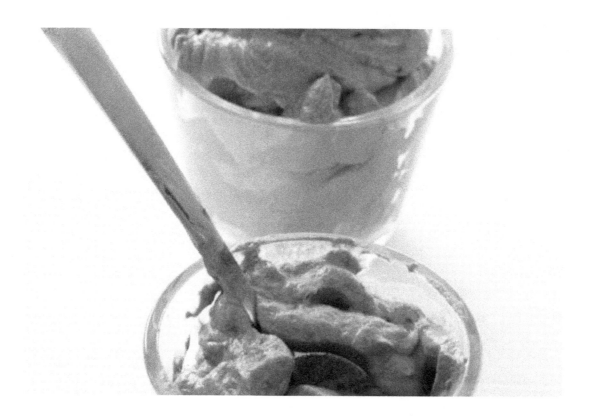

KETO SMALL APPLIANCE RECIPES

48. SLOW COOKER CHICKEN PROVENCAL

Ingredients

For 4 servings

- 1 eggplant, cut into 1-inch chunks
- 4 chicken thighs
- 1 tbsp olive oil
- 4 bacon slices, chopped
- 1 zucchini, cut in chunks
- 1 red chili, minced
- 2 cups passata
- 3 cloves garlic, minced
- 1 red onion, cut in wedges
- ½ cube chicken stock, crushed
- 1 tsp mixed herb seasoning
- ¼ cup chopped parsley

Directions

Total Time: approx. 8 hours 25 minutes

1. Warm the olive oil in a skillet over medium heat and fry the bacon until it is browned and crispy, about 4 minutes.

2. Add the chicken, red chili, red onion, eggplant, zucchini, and garlic and sauté for 5-6 minutes.

3. Remove to your slow cooker.

4. Pour in the passata, 1 cup of water, chicken stock cube, and mixed herbs seasoning.

5. Stir the ingredients lightly with a spoon, close the lid, and cook them for 8 hours on Low.

6. Once ready, open the lid and stir in the parsley. Dish the chicken with sauce and veggies into a serving bowl and serve it with some creamy broccoli mash if desired.

Per serving:

- Cal 250
- Fat 10g
- Net Carbs 1g
- Protein 22g

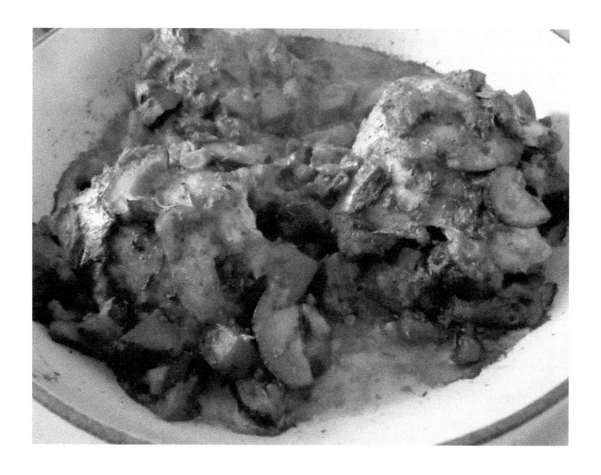

49. SLOW COOKER PORK & KRAUT

Ingredients

For 4 servings

- 1 lb pork tenderloin
- 1 (20 oz) sauerkraut, undrained
- ¼ cup butter
- Salt and pepper to taste

Directions

Total Time: approx. 8 hours 5 minutes

1. Put the pork in your slow cooker, pour the sauerkraut with its juice butter, 1 cup of water, salt, and pepper.
2. Cover the lid and cook the ingredients on Low for 8 hours.
3. Open the lid and use two forks to shred the tenderloin.
4. Also, add some water if the mixture is dry, and stir it with a spoon.
5. Serve the pork with mashed turnips and some steamed rapini if desired.

Per serving:

- Cal 258
- Fat 15g
- Net Carbs 7.5g
- Protein 22g

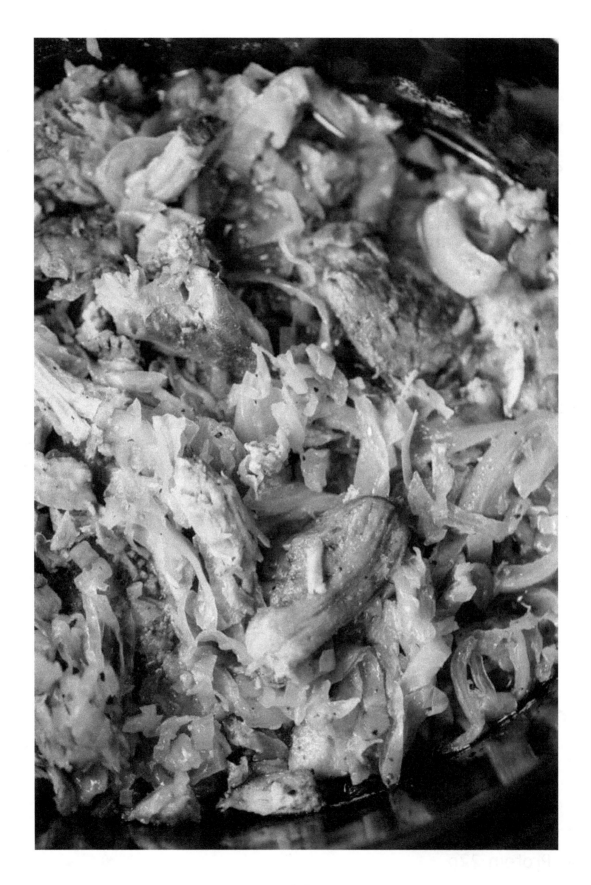

50. SLOW COOKER CHICKEN CACCIATORE

Ingredients

For 4 servings

- 1 cup sliced Cremini mushrooms
- 1 ½ lb chicken thighs, boneless
- 2 ½ tbsp olive oil
- Salt and pepper to taste
- 1 cloves garlic, minced
- 1 tsp rosemary
- 1 yellow onion, chopped
- 1 ½ cup crushed tomatoes
- 1 ½ tsp balsamic vinegar
- 1 green bell pepper, chopped
- 3 /4 cup chicken broth
- 3 /4 dry red wine
- 2 tbsp chopped parsley
- 2 tbsp grated Parmesan cheese

Directions

Total Time: approx. 4 hours 50 minutes

1. Put a skillet over medium heat and add two tablespoons of olive oil to warm. As it heats, season the chicken with salt and pepper and brown it on both sides for 6 minutes in total. Transfer the chicken to your slow cooker.

2. Then take the skillet over the heat and, use a paper towel to wipe it, return the skillet to heat, and heat the remaining olive oil. Pour in the onion and garlic and cook until softened

for 2 minutes, then add 1 tablespoon of balsamic vinegar. Cook until the vinegar reduces, 1-2 minutes. Pour the mixture into the cooker.

3. Add in the tomatoes, mushrooms, bell pepper, rosemary, chicken broth, and wine and stir. Close the lid and cook them on High mode for 4 hours. Serve the chicken garnished with chopped parsley and Parmesan cheese.

Per serving:

- Cal 228
- Fat 8g
- Net Carbs 4g
- Protein 28g

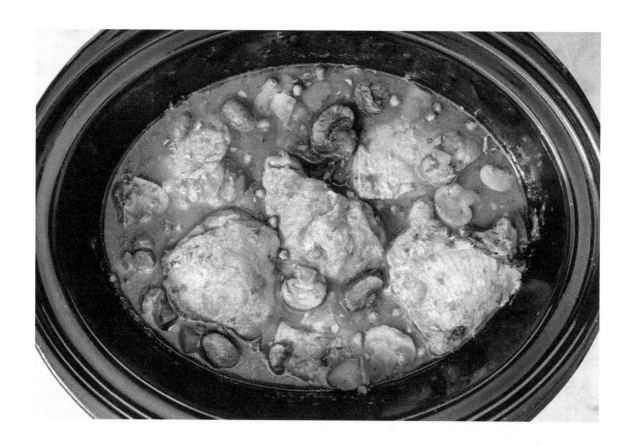

51. SLOW COOKER CHICKEN IN WINE SAUCE

Ingredients

For 6 servings

- 1 (14.5 oz) can cream of mushroom soup
- 2 (4 oz) cans mushrooms, drained
- 6 chicken breasts, boneless
- 1 /3 cup white wine
- 2 tbsp milk
- 2 tsp onion powder
- ½ tsp garlic powder
- 2 tsp dried parsley
- Salt and pepper to taste

Directions

Total Time: approx. 6 hours 10 minutes

1. In your slow cooker, pour the mushroom soup, mushrooms, white wine, milk, onion powder, garlic powder, and dried parsley.
2. Season with salt and pepper and stir it with a spoon.
3. Put the chicken in the sauce and use the spoon to cover the chicken with some of the sauce.
4. Close the lid and cook it on High for 4 hours.
5. Open the lid after and dish the chicken with the sauce into serving bowls.

6. Serve on a bed of zoodles or squash spaghetti if desired.

Per serving:

- Cal 226
- Fat 5.1g
- Net Carbs 1.8g
- Protein 38g

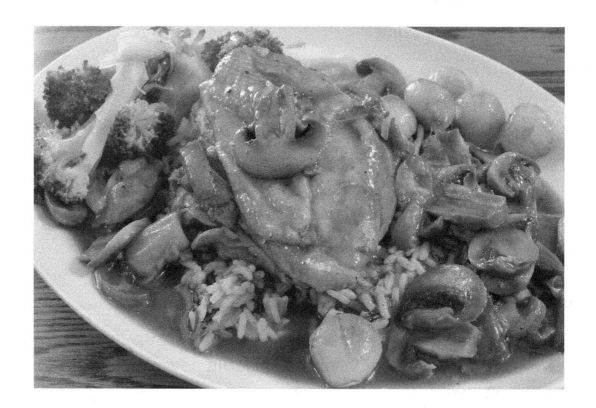

MEASUREMENTS & CONVERSIONS

	US STANDARD	US STANDARD (OUNCES)	METRIC (APPROXIMATE)
VOLUME EQUIVALENTS (LIQUID)	2 tablespoons	1 fl. oz.	30 mL
	¼ cup	2 fl. oz.	60 mL
	½ cup	4 fl. oz.	120 mL
	1 cup	8 fl. oz.	240 mL
	1 ½ cups	12 fl. oz.	355 mL
	2 cups or 1 pint	16 fl. oz.	475 mL
VOLUME EQUIVALENTS (DRY)	¼ teaspoon		1 mL
	½ teaspoon		2 mL
	1 teaspoon		5 mL
	1 tablespoon		15 mL
	¼ cup		59 mL
	⅓ cup		79 mL
	½ cup		118 mL
	⅔ cup		156 mL
	¾ cup		177 mL
	1 cup		235 mL
	2 cups or 1 pint		475 mL
	3 cups		700 mL
	4 cups or 1 quart		1 L
WEIGHT EQUIVALENTS	½ ounce		15 g
	1 ounce		30 g
	2 ounces		60 g
	4 ounces-		115 g
	8 ounces		225 g
	12 ounces		340 g
	16 ounces or 1 pound		455 g

	FAHRENHEIT (F)	CELSIUS (C) (APPROXIMATE)
OVEN TEMPERATURES	250°F	120°F
	300°F	150°F
	325°F	180°F
	375°F	190°F
	400°F	200°F
	425°F	220°F
	450°F	230°F